The
Widow's
&
Divorcee's
Handbook

Helps You Do
What He Used to Do

By Elaine Breakstone and Arlene Ball

Copyright © 2010 The Magni Group, Inc.

email: info@magnico.com

Website: www.magnico.com

ISBN: 978-1-882330-12-6

About the Authors

Ollie and Lainey were in the same boat as you. The attractive, slim, ex-vice-presidents of New York advertising agencies were baffled when, suddenly on their own, there were everyday things they didn't know how to do. Like building a fire, lighting the barbecue, turning off the outside water in Fall and turning it back on in Spring, flipping a mattress, dozens of easy tasks that HE used to do.

Think about it. Isn't that the way it happened?

Special Thanks to Special People

A word or two of thanks to the special people in our lives who helped make this book possible:

Bob Lelle, Bob Dempsey and Dick Lord who pushed us to write, edit, re-write, and re-write until we got it right.

Patty Barrington who gave us practical financial guidance and emotional support from Day One.

Pete D'Angelo at the local hardware store who edited our how-to's, gave our suggestions his blessing, and added his own tips and guidance. A man with an encyclopedic knowledge of nuts, screws and bolts and a love for what he does.

To friends, neighbors, family, and our ever present publisher Evan who encouraged our musings, stilled our anxieties, edited our manuscripts, and refused to let us be defeated.

Merci!

Lainey and Ollie

Table of Contents

Prologue

You're a smart lady, but suddenly YOU are a woman FLYING SOLO and, like a lot of other women in the same boat, without a clue of how to do the simplest of jobs. That's because HE always did them. He being YOUR husband, YOUR live-in partner, YOUR soul mate.

Let us give you simple to understand, easy-to-follow, step-by-step instructions for jobs we had to learn how to do the hard way.

Lainey and Ollie

How We Came to Write This Book

You never know when you're going to be called upon to take on a different role.

I was the working wife/mom/breadwinner. My husband handled the financials, dealing with the tradesmen, paying the bills, filling the role of general contractor/handyman. Happily, it was a role he liked and did well.

But fate dealt me a different hand, and I found myself faced with taking on a totally different role.

I had been caring for my husband at home helping him as best I could fighting the battle against lung cancer. Yes, I had help beyond nurses: a man who lived in and did the heavy lifting and light cooking while my husband battled the battle courageously.

Sadly, as was the case with my writing partner's husband, cancer won. Like most men, her husband Bill always had the answers to "how often do you change the air conditioner filters?" and "who checks out the flues at your house?" Like most women, Ollie's response was "I'll have to ask Bill."

And both of us were content to maintain this division of labor.

Until the big "C" entered our lives, and in what seemed like a mere blink of an eye, they were gone. There was no longer a man of the house, a Mr. Fix this and Fix that. And, like it or not, ready or not, we had to step up to the plate.

We're getting ahead of ourselves as we are want to do.

Man's Work.
Now It's a Job for a Woman!

It's not surprising that when you are called upon to do what is considered man's work, you think ... No way.

We urge you to bite the bullet, take a long, deep breath and face the task and TRY to do it as best you can.

For instance, I had watched my husband remove and replace the battery in one of the smoke alarms that had been squealing unmercifully at 2 in the morning.

The pattern was always the same:

> **Step 1**: Get ladder from laundry room.

> **Step 2:** Climb up and unscrew cover (alarm still squealing because most alarms have a mind of their own especially at 2 a.m.)

> **Step 3:** Remove battery. Beat alarm into submission.

> **Step 4:** Replace old battery with new one.

> **Step 5:** Re-connect cover and screw into place.

> **Step 6:** Light will show alarm is connected and working. Test beeper.

All of which sounds fast and easy even for a novice. Wrong. Just when I thought I had it down cold. Just when I was convincing myself that I could do what HE used to do, six months after he died, at 2 a.m. the smoke/fire alarm decided to make itself known. And I gave it a nod, and attempted to silence its ugly and very annoying squeal.

Thirty minutes of deafening noise and scorched temper later, I managed to pull the cover off and silence the intruder. Replacing the battery? Uh - uh. No back up batteries were available.

Murphy's Law. Most breakdowns happen after midnight.

Murphy's Law continued: Most single person households do not have back-up batteries on hand.

Note: See chapter on Back-ups Batteries, etc.

At 3:30 a.m. I decided that tomorrow I would call the alarm people and have them come to the rescue.

Five days and a sizable check later they fixed the alarm that had gone haywire, replaced a faulty key pad, and gave me a lesson on how to remove and replace the batteries. April lst (appropriate date) I made a pact with myself to overcome fear of failure performing simple tasks.

Trust me, they are simpler than you think. And as I subsequently found out: Simpler than HE made them out to be.

Ollie's Story and How She Found
the Right Answers at the Right Time

Meanwhile, my friend and fellow writer was having her own travails. Seems one wintry night Ollie was having a few couples over for cocktails. "It had been a whole year since Bill died, and I'd never used my fireplace. Didn't know where to begin. Who knew about laying logs?"

But this was a perfect night for a fire so she asked a guest (male of course) to do it. And HE did.

Except he forgot one important step: to open the flue!

Besides needing a major clean up and an equally costly paint job, Ollie now knows her alarm system's emergency phone number, and where the smoke alarms are located in her house. She also made up her mind to master the barbecue, plant the annuals, and has even put up shelves in her garage.

To put it succinctly, she now knows a lot of guy stuff!

An epiphany occurred.

Ollie realized that she was not alone; that there were thousands of women who find themselves helpless at doing what HE did around the house, tons more that haven't a clue about how to light a fire. She reminded me of the smoke alarm fiasco. Why not share our knowledge with them.

And so this book was born.

Today, we're pros at building a fire, fixing a leaky faucet and well versed in wines and bottle openings. We're proud of what we've learned. And eager to share our common sense knowledge and guidance with you.

This Book is not Just for Widows

Anyone who's on her own can find a wealth of information in these pages.

For instance, MBF (My Best Friend), and business partner had a mid-life crisis that, sad to say, affects thousands of women everywhere. The Big D. DIVORCE.

After 25 years of being what seemed on the surface happily married, she awakened one morning to find her husband had run off (figuratively and literally) with the 25 year old bookkeeper. And she thought he was out jogging!

Turns out that numbers were not the only thing the 25 year old was good at.

Suddenly single, MBF had to take on the role of chief bottle washer, carpenter, electrician and bill payer, along with being a mom and breadwinner. Totally overwhelmed, with only minor household skill aptitude, she turned to Ollie and me for help and advice and TLC. This was a lady who had never opened a ladder, never cleared a drain.

A light bulb went off. *Two* light bulbs!

Gosh, OLLIE AND I realized there must be hundreds, thousands of people just like My Best Friend that we can reach out to, inform, guide them through the maze of tasks HE used to do inside the house and out—and because we know the journey may not always be easy, give them an extra dollop of love and confidence.

Yes, MBF still has melt-down moments, but is fully committed to hanging in. Instead of just hanging on. She's repainted the porch, hung a chandelier in her dining room, and is seriously considering putting new tiles in the kitchen. Her Ex had been promising to do this for 3 years. TOO BUSY JOGGING was his excuse. Hmm.

Know that YOU are not Alone

The numbers speak for themselves.

More than 780,000 women lose their spouses each year. In 1998, there were 1,135,000 divorces. Countless couples separate each and every year.

Let's take a closer look at the statistics:

As of the 2005 census, there were 11.3 million widows in the U.S.

More than 780,000 women lose their spouses each year. By 2040, that number is estimated to grow to 1.25 million women.

80% of women live longer than their mates.

The average age of a widow is only 56! Surprised?

Nearly 50% of women over 65 are widowed.

25% are under 45. Surprised again?

Source: 2005 U.S. Census Bureau

Gaining Momentum
Talking to Women in the Same Place as We Were.

Armed with the knowledge that there are hundreds of thousands of women (700,000 widows are "born" every year, plus over a million couples separate or get divorced), Ollie and I set out to talk to women like us who are faced with starting over—whether they were widows, divorced or left solo when HE ran off with HER best friend.

What followed was a series of informal chats with friends, local book clubs, bridge groups, church groups, sharing our thoughts with others in the same place that we were. And they *are*.

We searched the internet to see if there were sources that could provide helpful information to women just like us. Not ones that required an engineering degree to understand, let alone follow. Nor sagas from financial gurus that required a MBA and a hefty check to receive mostly less than useful advice. And remarkably, there wasn't anything that came close to what we wanted to do.

Which made us realize: There is a crying need for a honest, straight-forward guide like this one. And written by women *to* women in the same place as we were.

And days and nights and weekends later, we arrived at this simple to understand, simpler to follow guide to doing what HE used to do.

We hope you will agree and that it will become your next best friend.

Happy and successful reading!

Elaine (lainey) Breakstone
Arlene (ollie) Ball

Building a Fire is Easy,
When You Know How

Let's begin with a strong male hold-out: Building a fire in the fireplace.

Nothing says MALE task faster than building a fire in the fireplace. And nothing labels YOU faster as being one of those "helpless" females.

Let's send that MALE task packing faster than you can say, "I can do it now!

Start with making sure fireplace is fairly tidy, and safely protected by a fire screen, away from drafts (close windows nearby), and flue is open. Check out necessary tools: poker to poke coals, grate to hold logs, optional bellows to fan fire, long matches, a heavy-duty mitt to prevent getting burned, a fire screen, a shovel to clean up debris, and a small fireplace broom to sweep up after.

> **Tip:** Most flues have markings that show when they're open or shut. Check out yours with a flashlight to be sure flue is open before you start. Otherwise, you may have two fires to put out!

Now the fire itself. Start with newspapers twisted as if you are wringing out a towel; 3 to 4 double pages will be sufficient. Lay newspapers on grate. Now add kindling wood (smaller easy-to-burn pieces of wood available at the local hardware or gardening store), and top these off with 3-4 logs real or store bought, easy starter logs. Now light fire with LONG matches. If your fireplace has glass doors, close them. If it doesn't, place fire screen at opening to contain fire in fireplace.

Enjoy!

As logs burn, you can use fireplace poker (long metal piece that is part of a fireplace set) to make sure you've got a good, healthy fire. Keep an eye on fire, and add new logs as others burn off.

And make sure to close the flue when fire has burned down.

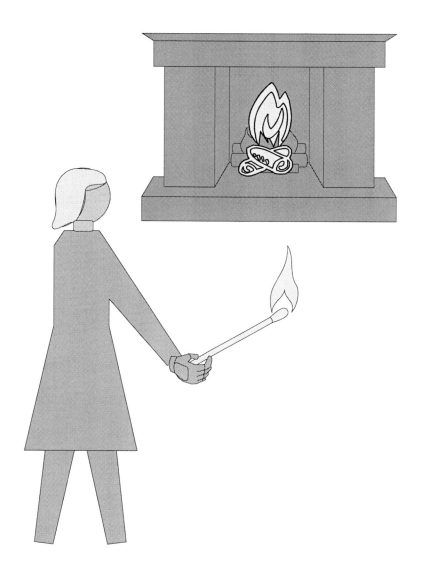

Fireplace Tools.
Part of HIS Building-a-Fire Ritual; Now Part of YOURS.

You probably never gave them a second glance, but part of the building a fire ritual that was always HIS job are fireplace tools.

They come in all shapes and sizes. Beyond being decorative, they are extremely useful. Here's a run-down:

> **Poker:** Vital to keeping the fire going. You use it to give the fire needed oxygen. Master this action and you will be the master of building a fire.

> **Tongs:** For adding logs to the fire. For moving logs around to keep the fire going. For looking totally in control of the situation.

> **Bellows:** To fan fire, keep it alive.

> **Shovel:** To remove ashes.

> **Broom:** Ditto above and keeps fireplace clean.

> **Stand:** An added flourish to your fireplace. Keeps tools neatly and attractively in one place.

> **Log carrier:** For carrying fresh logs from outside inside. Keeps you and your home neat.

> **Note:** There is absolutely nothing wrong with buying the ready-to-go logs that give great fire and are available in your local supermarket. They are often known as Sterno logs, and they do work.

> **Note:** But once you get the hang of doing it, building a fire the long way is empowering, very empowering.

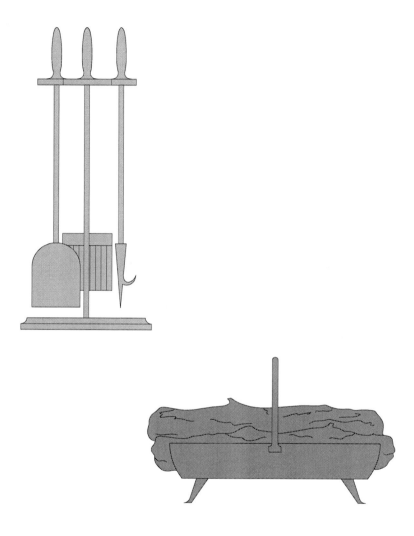

The Mystery of Opening a Bottle of Wine Solved Here

It all boils down to one small rule: the simpler the opener, the better! At one time I was the owner of a whole drawer full of esoteric openers. All of which I hadn't a clue how to use them. I tried the screw pull, the rabbit, even the estate model. No luck. Then I found an old-fashioned wing-type opener in the back of the drawer. Problem solved.

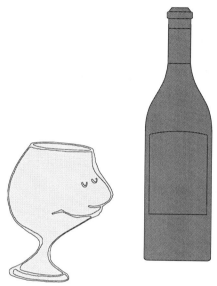

1. Hold opener in your left hand and place metal spiral (hence, the name corkscrew) into middle of cork.

2. Twist top. Two side wings will "fly" up as the cork moves up.

3. When wings are all the way up, push them down using two hands to bring cork all the way up and out of the bottle.

As you know, entertaining is hard without a man to help. This will be one less thing to worry about. Besides, all sommeliers have to start somewhere.

Tip #1: Open red wine 30 minutes before you plan to serve it. They say it lets the wine "breathe" …whatever that means. White wine? Chill first, open, and pour.

Tip #2: Left-over wine? Hardware stores carry small packages of rubber Stoppers ($6 or $7). They last a long time, and work great. White wine should be put in the fridge. And if you have left-over red, it will retain its body and taste a few days longer when it's refrigerated.

Tip #3: Left-over wine is great poured into a stew you're making.

HIS Tool Kit:
What to Keep and What to Pitch

It was HIS and his alone. Now it's your turn to know the difference between a Philips head screwdriver and a regular screwdriver.

First of all, unless it's big and too heavy to carry around, keep the tool box. You need an organized place for screws, nuts, bolts and everything in between.

> **Note:** See SOURCES for tools for women, tool kits, etc. at the end of this chapter. You may decide you want your own tools, etc.

Now comes the hard part. What to keep and what not to.

Here's a list of basics and why you need them:

> **A Phillips head screwdriver.** It's the one with grooved ends so you can use the right setting to do the job.

> **A flat head screwdriver.** They come in a variety of shapes and sizes. If you decide to start with two, a narrow and a wider head you'll do fine. The narrow head is useful for drawer and cabinet pulls, door hinges, door knobs and handles, switch plates, etc. The wider head for other household jobs.

> **Note:** Alternate choice would be a screwdriver with interchangeable heads.

> **Nails of various sizes and weights.** Also hooks to hang pictures. These come with directions on how to use, and what weight you need for specific picture or wall hanging.

> **Screws of various sizes.**

A good 12 foot tape measure, preferably the one that you can pull out, fasten, measure, then release. Colorful, lightweight ones can be found in our Sources for Tools for Women section.

Duct tape. Essential for temporary and semi-permanent first aid.

Pliers. Regular and needle nose

Hammer, a good one. And there are sources for Hammers for Women. See our Sources for Tools for Women Section in back.

Most practical and popular is the claw hammer appropriately named because its head is shaped like a claw which is also useful for removing nails. Weight should be between 16 and 24 ounces. If HIS IS HEAVY AND KLUTZY, TOSS IT OUT

Wrenches. A set of open and box-end wrenches.

Allen wrenches. These L-shaped tools don't look like wrenches at all. Come in sets or sold individually.

Utility and putty knife you can use for a variety of household tasks.

Hand saw.

Paint can key. Absolute must. Once you've tried to open a paint can with something other than this, you'll know why it's an absolute must.

Power drill. More and more women are finding that this belongs in a women's tool kit. Today they come light in weight and manageable. See SOURCES at end of this chapter.

Safety glasses. You may not have thought of this, but safety glasses are essential to home repairing. Manufacturers are now making them in lightweight materials and in shapes to fit your face.

Tools for Women—A New and Handy Idea

Because today more and more women are handling the handyman role, savvy manufacturers have tools and tool boxes and tool belts designed by women *for* women.

Lighter in weight, configured to fit a woman's hand, these are worth seeking out. They even come in pink! See SOURCES for Tools for Women at the end of this chapter.

Now what do you do with the rest of the "stuff" he's accumulated. Unless you are expecting to set up housekeeping for two in the near future, donate it to a neighbor, or pass it onto one of your kids (grown up variety), or give to a local charity.

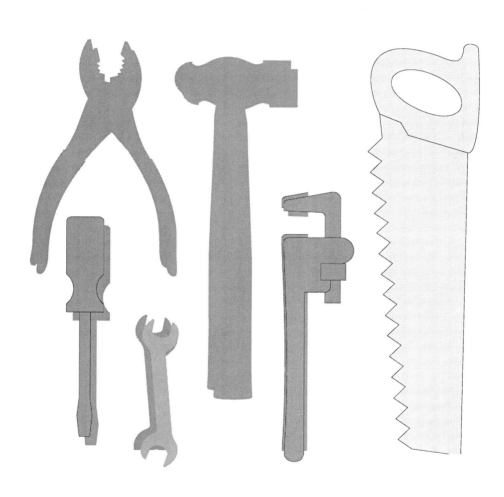

Sources for Tools for Women

BarbaraK Tools for Women

A former general contractor and single mom who has a full line of tools for women designed to be lightweight, easy to use, dependable. Line includes pliers, screwdrivers, tape measures, hammers, and a roadside emergency tool kit. Plus cordless power tools, a cordless screwdriver and a cordless drill/driver. BarbaraK also has a starter tool box for women

> On line at: **www.BarbaraK.com**. - Check out Barbara's Way for dozens of suggestions for home fix-its.

> **www.Sears.com**

> **www.GirlyLock.com** - Tools specifically made for women. Many come in pink.
> Check out their cute hard hat in pink!

> **www.helpinghandtools.net** - Check out Latitude Tools for women video on their website. Awesome!

> **Ladies Tool Zone** - Offers lightweight tools in pink and other feminine colors. Here you'll find an 87 piece tool set for women for less than $30.

> **Grip Tools** - Offers 10 and 30 piece tool kits for women with all the basic hand tools for $40. The 30 piece set includes nails, screws and picture hangers.

> **DeWalt** - Manufactures tools for women, designed lighter, easier to handle.

> **Makita** - A heavy weight in the high quality power tool industry; makes a smaller cordless drill designed for women. Lightweight, fits woman's hands.

> **Black & Decker** - Offers the Smartdriver cordless screwdriver, designed for women.

Tomboy Tools - Offers household tool kits, garden tools for women, auto tool kits. Check out their "body pocket", a tool belt for women holding basic household tools designed for women. As the market has expanded and more and more women are doing home repairs, Tomboy Tools has added dry wall, painting, plumbing, molding, tiling tool kits for women.

On line at: **www.TomboyTools.com** - An intriguing website dedicated to educating women about home repairs.

Grandma Purples - Household and garden tools for women

Home Depot - Check the yellow pages or on-line at **www.Homedepot.com** They even offer classes for do-it-yourself-ers. FREE! You can also check out their website.

Lowe's - Check the yellow pages or on line for a Lowe's nearest you. Some offer FREE classes for do-it-yourself-ers. You can also check out their website. **www.lowes.com**

Target Stores - Check out their website www.target.com for a store near you, and to see if they offer the tools you need. They also offer a pink roadside assistance tool kit which includes jumper cables, pliers, adjustable wrench and other necessities.

Pink Tool Box! - From the UK. Contains the basics: hammer, pliers, screwdriver, Allen wrenches, scissors, level, knife adjustable wrench, tape measure and more in a handy, lightweight pink box.

Oxo Good Grips - Available at Lowe's

Stanley - Offers a 13 ounce hammer

Workforce - Offers Color Rules Tape Measure with a soft grip handle

Metabo Corp. - Offers a 1 1/2 pound power drill that packs 80 pounds of torque. Check their website at: www.metabousa.com

Safety Glasses - AOSafety and Echo offer designs that fit a woman's face. Available at most home improvement centers.

Sources for Tool Belts for Women

Girl Gear Industries - Offers both belts and pouches for holding tools

Grip Tools

Girly Lock - Offers female tool belts as well as hard hats, safety glasses, and carpenters' pencils.

Take a Breather

Pour yourself a cup of tea or a cup of coffee or a nice cold glass of lemonade.

Now put your feet up, and RELAX.

Know that you're on top of it, YOU can do it, fix what HE used to fix and do it faster, and maybe better.

You're in charge now. And we're proud of you.

For more help, advice on how to cope with everyday fix-its…keep on reading…

Plumbing: Be Prepared.
The Tools YOU Need in Case Something Goes Wrong

FIRST, A quick run-down on essential plumbing tools. HE probably had them. YOU should, too.

For pipes: Adjustable pipe wrench to give you a tight grip on pipe fittings.

For w.c. aka toilet: Plunger aka "the plumber's friend." Will eliminate most clogs by creating a vacuum and allowing natural pressure to free the water flow.

For tub and sink: Plumber's snake, the best tool to unclog a clogged drain. By twisting and turning it, you un-clog the clog.

Adjustable and open-end wrenches. Drain fittings tend to be very tight; an open end wrench will provide a tighter grip.

NEXT, What can go wrong, and how to fix it:

The Toilet: Friend or Foe

It's a dirty job, but someone has to do it. And now it's YOU.

I'm talking about the toilet, and when it's stuffed up, it's a mess to deal with.

Yes, you can call a plumber and wait and wait and wait. And pay and pay. Or you can dive in (figuratively speaking) and try and fix it yourself.

High on the must-have-on-hand list is a plunger. Buy, if HE didn't already have one, the up market "biggie" that has a large rubber head on it. Mine has a bulbous, layered head that looks something like this:

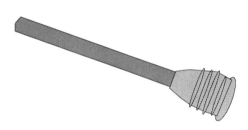

Often called "the plumber's friend", this "biggie" helps build suction as you work it up and down inside the toilet bowl. The more suction you can work up, the easier and faster the toilet will be running smoothly again.

Next, plunge slowly. Push down, hold for a few minutes, then release. This creates suction that hopefully will release what is "stuck" below. Wait a few minutes and try again.

If waste goes down drain, lucky you, flush toilet, let water refill bowl, then flush again. In case you didn't realize it, this is also an excellent exercise for developing upper arm strength. Think Jennifer Aniston biceps.

If success doesn't happen, repeat process. Or consult hardware store about special products that "un-stuff " stuffed up toilets.

For example, Pete at our local hardware store recommends products such as RID-X, that will break up toilet paper and debris in your septic tank. Use regularly to avoid future problems.

If all else fails, call a plumber.

IMPORTANT: Never ever pour drain opener into a toilet. It dissolves the wax ring that mounts the toilet, and will cause your toilet to leak, and you're looking at major damage and major expense.

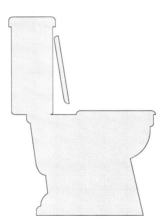

Quick Fixes for the W.C.
Or
Don't Let a Broken Flapper Flip You Out

Just when you thought everything was running smoothly, the w.c. keeps running non-stop. And YOU, smart lady, can handle it without a frantic call to the plumber.

First and foremost, turn OFF the water. Do so by reaching behind or under the toilet bowl, making sure to tighten handle securely.

Next, check out flapper (see illustration). It may be old or damaged or both so it no longer seals correctly. Clue here is water that keeps running in the toilet tank. If it is worn out, replace it at local hardware store or plumbing supply place.

> **Tip:** If you haven't done so already, introduce yourself to the hardware store, home improvement center or plumbing supply place "helper". Even biggies like Lowe's and Home Depot have seasoned employees who know their way around the plumbing section. This man who is soon to become your best friend can and will show you how easily you can re-place this piece.

Replace flapper, open pipe to turn water ON, and begin flushing to your w.c.'s content.

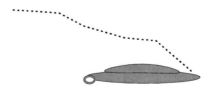

The Kitchen Sink: Sink or Swim!

Leaks under the sink often happen without any warning. Drips become puddles. Puddles become streams.

Again, don't panic. Chances are the leak is coming from a missing or worn-out washer inside the pipe. Once you turn off the water in the pipe, you can unscrew it, and replace the worn out washer.

Visit the man who by now you should have a warm relationship with: your local hardware store person. He can provide the right washer for that pipe, and that drip, drip, drip will go bye-bye-bye.

Tip: If you've got plastic pipes, you're in luck as they last longer and are easier to fix.

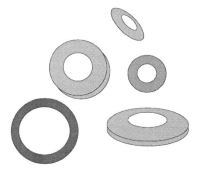

Leaky Faucet?
Make that Drip, Drip, Drip Go Bye-Bye

Water torture takes on a whole new meaning when, no matter how you tighten the handle, the faucet continues to drip, drip, drip. Ignore it, and trust me, that drip will turn into drops, and drops will turn into a stream.

Shut off water. Knobs are usually under the sink to do this. Remove screw CARE-FULLY with a flat headed screwdriver (see chapter on Tools for Women for help) Do so by turning screw counter-clockwise. This will release handle.

Underneath handle is a metal fixture that can be pulled or unscrewed out (turning it counter-clockwise). Now look inside this piece and you'll find a rubber washer, round and what is supposed to keep the water out, by now torn, ripped or com-pletely gone.

IMPORTANT: This sad washer is what you take to the hardware store to get a replacement.

You may also want to take the piece the washer went into just to be sure you get the right washer. Be a sport...buy a few back-ups and keep them in YOUR tool chest, marked.

Put washer back into metal fixture, and hook up. Turn on hot and cold water. Slowly.

> **Tip:** To protect against tools scratching metal, wrap pipe and/or faucet with cloth.

Clogged Shower Head? No Problem

You've probably noticed that things you take for granted can suddenly throw you a curve. One day the shower is your friend, delivering water graciously and in abundance. Be grateful.

But just when you thought everything was going smoothly, Old Faithful begins to slow down to a spray. Soon, there's just a trickle of water. The cause: most likely, calcium and lime deposits in your water.

Once again, YOU can step in and become Ms. Fix-it.

Here's how: Make sure water is fully turned off. Next, unscrew shower head. You may need a wrench to get a good hold on the head and/or the pipe holding the shower head in place. Remove the head and carefully clean inside. A toothbrush that has seen better days is a handy helper for digging out grime and mineral deposits.

Your local hardware store can also suggest a specific drain/shower head cleaner. One that cleans, breaks down calcium and lime deposits, eliminates rust stains.

Rinse thoroughly and replace. If you're wet and sticky or wet and sticky and dirty, now's the time to test your shower head.

Tip: I use toothpicks or Q-tips to poke through holes and clear "gunk" out of stuffed up shower heads.

HE Fixed the Dripping Shower Head in a Jiffy. Can YOU?

Now YOU know how to fix a CLOGGED shower head. But what about the reverse: the one that drips and drips?

No problem for YOU now. Using pliers, unscrew shower head from its pipe. Check inside pipe: there should be a rubber or plastic washer. Probably worn out, damaged, sorely in need of replacement.

Replace washer. As discussed above, take the damaged washer to your local hardware/home improvement center, and a buy new one (back-ups as well).

After you replace washer, seal connection on the pipe with a pipe sealer or heat resistant (teflon) tape. Screw shower head back in by hand. Do not over tighten.

Now turn on shower for two minutes.

Shut off. Wait an hour.

Now check to see if shower is still dripping. Job well done!

> **NOTE:** IF YOU SEE CRACKS OR WEAKNESS IN SHOWER HEAD, IT MAY BE TIME TO GET A NEW ONE.

Happily, you will be ahead of the game, knowing how to change the washer.

Stuffed Up Drains. What a Pain!

Pretty soon, you'll be hanging out a shingle: The Plumbing Lady Lives Here!

Let's start with how to prevent the stuffed up drain in the first place. Do NOT under any circumstances, brush or comb hair over the drain in the sink or shower. Same goes for other "stuff" like dental floss, tissue, hair pins, safety pins, etc., and my personal nemesis, rice that HE used to put down the kitchen sink. Stuff like that belongs in the garbage, in the compactor or the disposal unit if you have one.

BUT no matter how careful you are, nasty materials can get thrown in and clog the smooth operation. Take action immediately. Repeat. Take action immediately.

Visit your favorite hardware store. By now, you're probably on a first name basis with this person. HE will recommend a variety of liquid or powder remedies, and how to use them. Nine times out of 10, they work.

Most likely, his top recommendation will be the plumber's snake; if HE didn't own one, YOU should. Flexible yet firm, this genius "snakes" itself around as you turn it, allowing it to reach down into the pipe and unclog what's clogged.

What a smart lady. That's YOU!

> **Tip:** From one of the ladies in our focus groups: Her EX'S solution was to drop three Alka-Seltzer tablets down the drain. Add a cup of white vinegar, let sit 10 minutes, then flush with hot water. WE found the plumber's snake a better solution.

OOOPS! Down the Drain.
But Now it's Retrievable...by YOU!

Somehow or other, guys seem to know about plumbing. I didn't ... until now. And NOW I don't have to call a plumber when something to do with water goes awry.

Are you nodding, "yes, sounds like me... I would fail Plumbing for Beginners if I were up against the hot pipes." Don't give up. Listen up. Here's a simple, short lesson that will save you money, time, aggravation and that expensive call to the plumber.

At one time or another, all of us, well almost all of us, drop something down the bathroom sink. Often something valuable like a ring. Next time this happens, don't panic, simply follow these easy steps to getting that precious keepsake back.

Get out your wet/dry shop vacuum. Do NOT use a regular vacuum; water and electricity are NOT a safe combination.

NEXT, put a panty hose over the nozzle, turn on the vac and hold it over the sink's drain opening. Like magic, your missing valuable will appear. You should also run water in the sink for a few minutes after.

> **Note:** Don't own a wet/dry shop vacuum? Invest in one. They run about $30 and can be found at your local hardware store or home improvement center.

> If you've ever had the water pipe to your fridge's ice maker burst and cause a flood in the kitchen, you'll count your blessings you own a wet/dry shop vacuum.

> If you've ever had a wet basement, you'll be relieved you own this indispensable helper.

Now, smartie, when something drops down the drain, don't panic. Rescue it! Cause YOU know YOU can do it! And NOW YOU know how to do it.

Opening a Stubborn Lock
or Worse Yet, a Lock that Freezes

It seems to happen when YOU least expect it. You put the key in the lock to the front door; your other hand is holding a bag of groceries.

Despite the tugging and jiggling, the lock refuses to open. You try again; again, nothing. You examine the key to be sure you're using the right key. Yes. But again, the door remains locked.

Fortunately for you, your neighbor has an extra key, and a more determined approach to unlocking doors and the door finally opens. Your neighbor also recommends a tube of graphite available at the home improvement center or the hardware store. You seem to remember that HE had a similar spray in his tool chest.

This should immediately send up a red flag. STOP what you're doing right now, and get yourself to the hardware store or home improvement center and BUY a graphite spray/powder. And put it in YOUR tool chest.

Here's how these sprays work: Spray some graphite powder into the key slot and work the key in and out. You might have to do this several times, but door will unlock. MAGIC!

Note: We recommend using graphite to loosen key from lock rather than using a machine lubricant oil. Less chance of dirt getting in and clogging opening.

Note: The lock itself may be worn and beyond repair. If so, get a locksmith to install a new one.

Next, what about a lock that freezes in winter? Our hero at the hardware store recommends a special spray that unfreezes frozen locks in a jiffy. Insert the tip into the lock and press liquid into the opening. Open sesame! It might be smart to keep an extra can of this spray in your car or in your house. It may come in handy when temperatures drop, and your car's parked outside.

Hinges that Squeak? EEEEK

This is an easy one. Oil them with a lubricating oil (see your hardware store or home improvement store for suggestions). Popular one that HE used was WD-40 spray. Pure genius. Keep it handy especially in hot sticky weather.

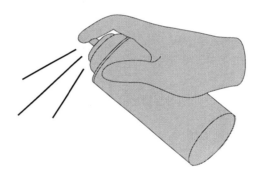

A Sliding Door that Gets Stuck/Won't Slide

Doors to decks, doors to patios, especially the ones that are supposed to slide easily back and forth do get stuck. And more often when you force them, come off their tracks. HE knew how to keep them sliding easily back and forth.

Now it's YOUR turn to figure out what to do. First, clean the track on top and bottom with a clean rag. Now spray the channels with a lubricating spray (found at the local home improvement center or hardware store). Wipe down with a rag. Now try that stubborn door. Easy, right?

If the door has come off its track (screen doors are notorious for doing this), hold it up to top part of door, place on track, then wiggle bottom part onto track. This may take a few attempts before you succeed, but keep at it. Like they say, if at first you don't succeed....

Note: There are products called Sliding Door Lubricants that look like a large wax crayon. You rub them back and forth in the track and like magic, the door slides easily!!

The Fuse Box
HE Knew Where it Was. Do YOU?

The fuse box was very much an unknown...until NOW!

And let us reassure YOU right now that we are NOT under any circumstances urging you to learn how to change fuses or become a master electrician. Our recommendation here is to delegate heavy duty electrical jobs to a legitimate electrician, even if YOUR significant other helped here.

BUT it is important to know that inside the fuse box are circuit breakers connecting to light sources. And when there is an outage, YOU should know where the fuse box is located, and what switch to "switch on or off".

If HE didn't label the circuit breakers, when the electrician comes, have him label them or help YOU label them. This could come in handy when you lose electricity, and the utility company tells you what to do in person or over the phone.

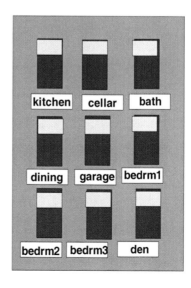

The Ice Maker Decided to Take a Vacation. Now What?

Admit it. Most of us are spoiled having that wonderful invention, the ice maker, in our fridge. And some of us are really spoiled having one that delivers a choice of water, cubes or shaved ice without having to open the door.

WHOA...just when you thought that wonderful invention was popping out crystal clear, perfectly shaped cubes, it decides to konk out.

Sure you could resort to those trays that came with the old clunker. Or you could try and fix it yourself. First, check the manufacturers' handbook that came with the fridge which gives helpful advice on how to fix minor problems.

> **Note:** See chapter on GETTING ORGANIZED which discusses need for organizing documents, warranty books, manufacturers handbooks, etc. Keeping manuals for all your appliances in one handy place is a very smart idea. Was HE that organized? Chances are HE WASN'T.

Often ice makers are clogged from dis-use. You're away for a week or more, and you forgot to tell the ice maker. Cubes build up and eventually the ice maker STOPS. OR you are left with one solid block of ice that is of no use whatsoever.

SO MAKE SURE YOU TURN OFF ICE MAKER WHEN YOU ARE AWAY. AND TURN IT BACK ON WHEN YOU RETURN.

> **Tip:** Most ice makers inside fridge have a metal bar on the side of the bucket that collects ice. And most have clearly visible markings that tell you the ice maker is on or off. Check it out to make sure it's ON before you invite 20 people over for drinks and a barbecue.

I Know How to Change the Filter in my Coffee Maker. But What about the other Ones: the Central Heating, the Air Conditioners?

IF you're like most of us, you do not spend a lot of time in the basement where the water heater and the central heating and AC units live. And for years, HE was the one who checked on what needed to be done each season, like changing the filter periodically to keep everything running smoothly.

You may even have a service that comes every six months to clean, refresh and restart your central heating and air conditioning units. You're ahead of most of us.

However, if YOU'RE in charge of making sure air, heat, gas, oil is running smoothly, here are tips to help ease the task:

Change filters every season. It's smart. It's cost efficient. And it's easier than you think.

Remove old filter. Most slide out easily. Take that with you to your local hardware or building/gardening/home supply store because there are dozens of sizes available.

We suggest you buy several to keep on hand. Amazing isn't it, how dirty yours looks? Amazing, too, how much money you can save heating your home, condo, or apartment with clean filters in place.

If you have a regular service contract with a heating professional, checking your heating unit, replacing filters are part of their 6 month service contract. These contracts aren't cheap, but if you've ever found yourself in mid-winter when it's colder inside than out, you'll appreciate the added insurance of knowing they're on call 24/7.

Window Air Conditioners

Air conditioning units also need to have their filters changed. Stuff can clog, slow down and burn out motors in a wink. As with a central unit, it's important to change filters every season to keep unit sending out fresh, clean air. Remove filters before summer, take to hardware store or home improvement center, and replace with fresh ones. Again, like filters for central air units, these come in many different sizes so it's good to take the old one with you. You may want to keep several on hand as back-ups.

Again, unless you are presently co-habitating with an MIT graduate, it's money well spent to have service contracts on air conditioners, and other major appliances. Our philosophy here is you're ahead of the game having insurance against what could and usually does go wrong.

Question: Where do you keep the use and care booklets and warranty information for your appliances? Check chapters on Safekeeping.

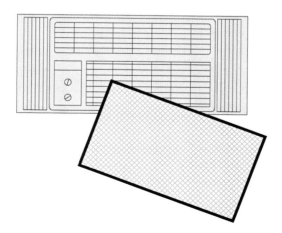

The Cold Facts about the Water Heater

You probably know where the water heater is…in the basement. You also know that up to now, it was His job to oversee it when it worked. And when it didn't.

It's time you knew the cold facts about the water heater. Like other major appliances, the water heater comes with an owner's manual (those books you stuff in a drawer and never look at again). You will get a general overview of the unit and how it works. Next, check out the unit itself.

Usually on the front there's a round knob or lever that regulates water temperature. Which you can lower or raise depending upon how you like your shower or bath temperature. Usually this same knob/lever or one nearby is labeled "vacation". This is a valuable accessory; use it when you are going to be away days, weeks. It's energy saving, cost saving.

And don't forget to adjust it back to your normal temperature when you return.

You'll also find a pressure release valve that releases air bubbles that can build up inside the heater itself. It's a good idea to release these air bubbles every few months to keep your water heater looking and feeling "hot". What a smart lady you've become!

But, you say, what do you do when it shakes, rattles and rolls and refuses to provide hot water? My solution b.t.g. (before the guide) was to think that, like snow, it will go away by itself. Reality check: it doesn't .

Now — before you call the expensive (and probably sunning himself in Saint Barth's at this very moment) technician, check the manual for service centers near you. Also, check the water heater itself; installers generally leave an emergency repair/service number.

> **Tip:** Keep a list of service providers next to your phone or other easily accessible location. Also see section on List Keeping and Service Providers.

Living Life Solo Fact of Life: Nine out of 10 appliances (Example: Smoke Alarms) break down after midnight.

Saving Money:
Something HE Realized. Now, so Should YOU

Now that you're into doing what used to be HIS jobs, YOU should feel emotionally rewarded AND financially rewarded. Honest! Repairing minor plumbing problems, doing simple repairs inside and outside your house can and will save you hundreds, maybe thousands of dollars.

And whether you're aware of it or not, this is positively, absolutely, no doubt about it, guaranteed to put a great big smile on your face.

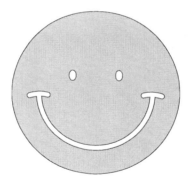

Flipping a Mattress: As Easy as Flipping Jacks

They don't call it man-ual labor for nothing. Turning a mattress is and always has been a man's job in our house. Now, since man's work is woman's work, what do YOU do?

Have a big breakfast or double up on weights at the gym? Perhaps.

Attack the task at hand. Actually two handed. Strip the bed. Lift the top RIGHT hand corner leaning against it with your whole body. Pull it towards you, moving it off the frame, keeping it against your body. Release. Do NOT pull it fully off the bed because that is where you will be sleeping from this moment on.

Take the bottom LEFT hand side, lift it towards you, leaning against it with your body and rolling it toward top left hand side. You should now have a half folded mattress or facsimile thereof.

Now keep maneuvering mattress until it's fully turned.

Make bed and take a nap or take a nap and make bed.

Open Sesame!
(Opening Lids on Jars,
Clamshell Packaging)

Long ago and far away, when I was having major trouble getting a lid off a jar, I I'd simply say, "Honey, can you please help me?" Done!

Alas, it's a different story now that HE's gone. I clench my teeth and put a towel around the top, or grab a knife or scissors or whatever. Once I even called the police. Honest! At wit's end, sick in bed, feeling horrible with a virus and unable to open an antibiotic, I called 911! Explaining I did not have an emergency but rather a problem, a kindly dispatcher said she'd have a police person on his driving rounds stop by. An hour later, my medicine container was open, and I told a very sweet guy a contribution would be on its way to the PAL.

My pharmacist now has a huge note in his computer that I do NOT need child proof tops. I, meanwhile, have found ways to open the "un-openables" and would like to share them with you:

1. Latex dishwashing gloves. Most of us have them stashed under the sink. They will give you a non-slip grip that should get a tight lid off every time.

2. Or, wrap a rubber band around the top, and it will give you enough grip to work the lid loose.

Now, let's get off jars and onto that impossible thing called "clamshell"... a very popular form of packaging. It is everywhere. A heavy, clear plastic, tightly sealed wrapping that allows you to see what's inside.

For example, hair brushes come this way: Stapled or sealed to a piece of cardboard with this clamshell plastic wrapping. Attractive visually. But almost impossible to open...unless YOU know what you are about to read:

Take a manual rotary can opener. Turn over the package to the back. Clamp the opener on the top right of the package and cut around the package.

Not as good as a guy. But what is?

Note: Stores that carry kitchen helpers may offer a mechanical lid opener. However, our way is cheaper and probably more rewarding.

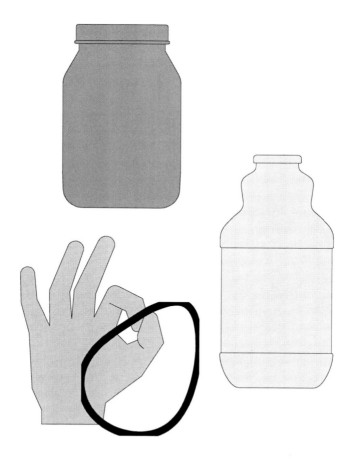

How to Hang a Picture:
The Dumb/Wrong Way vs. the Smart/Right Way

No, friend, YOU don't eyeball the wall and try a few nails here and there and hope for the best.

That is what we commonly refer to as the WRONG way!

Now the smart, right way...the way HE did it.

To begin, pictures are hung with bonafide picture hooks. Your local hardware store has them in all sizes. We said hooks. Not nails, not masking tape, hooks.

Now make sure you get the right picture hook for the weight of your picture. The reverse side of the hook package gives you weight restrictions, and often extra guidance. And don't be afraid to ask in the hardware store for help.

The simple 4-step "picture perfect" hanging technique:

1. Measure along the top of your picture frame and mark the halfway point with a pencil dot.

2. Hold the picture up where you want it on the wall and put a dot on the wall that corresponds with the dot you made on the top of the frame.

3. Turn the picture over, and gently pull the middle of the hanging wire towards the top of the picture and measure the distance between the top of the frame and where the wire is stretched to.

4. Mark off the same measurement from the dot on the wall...down towards the floor...and make another dot. That's where you hammer in your picture hanging hook.

Three pictures in a row: Follow same technique, allowing 3-4 inches of space between each picture, depending upon size of each one.

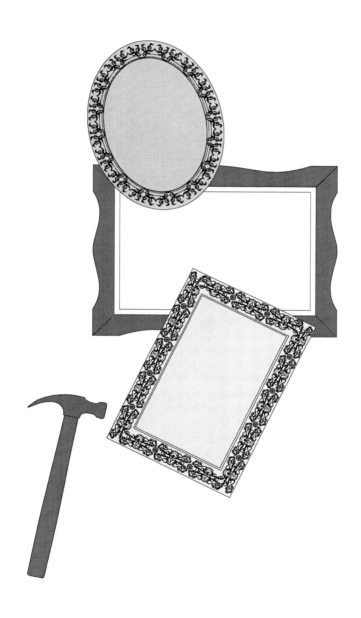

Light Bulbs 101

In my house, changing a light bulb was a guy thing. I just never did it. My turn came one night when my reading lamp went out. Hardly a challenge, I thought, until all I could find was a three-way bulb. I knew the lamp only had a one-way socket.

Now, can you put a three-way bulb (what we call regular or incandescent) into a one-way lamp? No one to ask. I thought maybe I could get a shock or blow out the lamp. But I went ahead, and no problem. After that, I decided to educate myself on lighting.

Here's why a 3-way bulb worked:

Inside a light bulb is a small wire called a filament that turns orangish and emits light when electricity is supplied to it. A 3-way bulb has two different filaments in it. One, a 50 watt filament, the other a 100 watt filament. If you had a three-way socket, it would have two bottom contacts, letting you turn on 50, 100 or both together for 150.

When you put your bulb in a one-way socket, which has just a single contact on the bottom, only one filament will turn on. It will be the 100 watt filament since it is the only one connected to the single center contact. Got it? If not read this again.

But let's get back to that empty box that should have been holding bulbs. Before you go out and buy anything, find out what type bulb is most efficient for your particular use. Your friend at the hardware store can bring you up to speed. Take some time investigating the inventory, and ASK questions.

But here's a speed course on the subject.

First, THE LANGUAGE. You know filaments. How about **lumens**? This is the word used to measure the light produced by a bulb.

Life. This is a guesstimate of the number of hours a bulb with last. Once you compare the life of different bulbs of the same wattage, you can figure out which bulb will work best for you in terms of color, how long they will last, and light output.

Watts. You know this, right? It is the standard measure of electricity.

Next, a few examples of different types of bulbs:

INCANDESCENT: The bulb you are probably most familiar with. They are inexpensive, and come in 15 to 150 watts. Your new found friend at the hardware store can give you an on-site run down of the different types: frosted, pastel, shatter resistant, energy saving, etc. Most commonly used for interior of your house.

Note: DON'T forget to buy back-ups. ALSO, see chapters on back-ups for batteries, bulbs, etc.

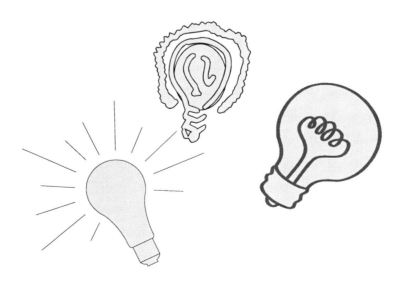

COMPACT FLUORESCENT. (CALLED CPL) Heads up! These are the most energy efficient of any kind of bulb. And we mean REALLY ENERGY EFFICIENT. They use 67% less energy than incandescent, and they last longer— up to 16 times longer! Initially they cost more, but because they last longer, they really end up costing less. Nice to know. Can be used in a standard fixture. Because of their extra long life, they work great in hard-to-reach places.

One caveat here: Sometimes, with legislation changing yearly, these may be difficult to dispose of. Check out your local rulings. For instance, in 2007, Congress passed an energy law that goes into effect in 2011, which could mean the end of inefficient incandescents. Research is being conducted to save the incandescent by matching the efficiencies of the CPL while keeping things people prefer about the popular incandescents, including its color.

A CHART TO CHECK OUT

Important to note here: Watts are not the same in these two types of bulbs. Here's a handy chart to help you compare them:

Incandescent	Compact Fluorescent
100 watts	25
75 watts	20
60 watts	13
40 watts	9

FLUORESCENT: You probably think of them as a linear light source, but they are also available in U-shape and circular. They last longer than incandescent lights and come in a range of colors...black for one.

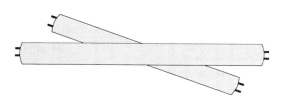

HALOGEN: Like most, these are more expensive than incandescent, but last three times longer and for the same amount of energy, you get 50% more light. Very fashionable as well; decorators love them.

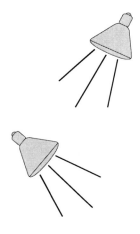

More About Lighting:
Don't Be in the Dark

I just learned something this past weekend and am thrilled with my new knowledge. A handy little tidbit that neither Lainey nor I knew, but it's a safe bet HE did.

For years, I assumed that the switch at the door to a small library in my home didn't work. I'd switch it on; nothing. Assuming it was non-functioning, I would grope around in the dark until I found a lamp inside the library I could click on. Right?

WRONG!

It took a friend with a keener knowledge of electric outlets 15 minutes to enlighten me. We went to each outlet in the room, plugged an adjacent lamp into each of its two sockets and then tried the switch. No luck, no luck, until Voila! The switch finally worked in one of the outlets. Hooray, now I could turn a light on from the entrance to the room.

I figured if one socket in an outlet didn't work with the switch, the other wouldn't. WRONG!

Now YOU know that only one socket is wired to the switch at the door. YOU just have to make the right connection.

End of indoor lighting lesson!

OUTDOOR LIGHTING:
Solar. Halogen Floodlights. Motion Detectors.

SOLAR lights: essential on paths and walkways, great for highlighting landscaping. Very efficient and inexpensive to put in because no wiring is needed. Powered by the sun, solar lights turn on automatically at dusk. Make sure they are placed in an area that gets some sunlight during the day. Otherwise, they will not store enough energy to provide light later in the day and night. Easy to change where you place them. And you can store them inside in winter if you prefer.

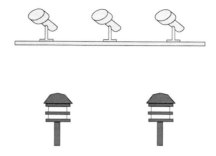

HALOGEN FLOODLIGHTS: Provide extra security outside your home. Medium efficiency. Can be screwed into standard outdoor floodlight fixtures.

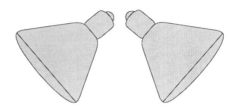

As we noted before, we suggest you visit your local hardware store and spend some time in the lighting department. Take a good look at everything, and talk with the sales person in charge. The one that's your new best friend now that you've lost the one you had all these years.

If you live in a house where deer live nearby, we suggest adding:

MOTION DETECTOR: Turns on with movement, frightening the deer. This works SOMETIMES. Remember, THE ONLY deer that are dummies are stuffed ones.

You'll find more information on Motion Detectors in the Home Security chapters.

Other useful information (YOU probably know this already but just in case):

Use energy saving fluorescent bulbs when and where you can.

Do NOT tighten bulbs when you screw them in. If they're too tight in the socket, they will burn out more quickly. HONEST!

Dimmer switches offer flattering lighting and save energy. It's like candle-light only smarter.

Energy Savers: Today a Must

Today, more than ever before, it's important to look for ways to save energy. HE probably was not as aware of them as YOU are today. WE offer a few suggestions that could help:

For starters:

Weather strip your doors and windows. If the draft from the front door, despite the storm door, feels like the Arctic, follow this easy to do weather-stripping.

Weather-stripping comes in rolls of tape with sticky backing. Found at the home improvement center or your local hardware store.

Before you begin, be sure the surfaces are clean. Dirt will prevent the sticky backing from sealing. Measure the surface you're intending to cover, i.e. inside of door or window. Lay the weather strip against it, unrolling it carefully so it will lie smooth and snug. Using scissors, cut the piece to fit, and press down, removing backing tape as you go.

This can make an amazing difference. And even if you live in an apartment, this is a smart idea. Drafts from halls and windows happen everywhere.

P.S. Cover and seal around window air conditioners to prevent leaks.

Other tips to save energy:

Make sure fireplace dampers are closed when you're not using the fireplace.

If you have ceiling fans, use them to keep heated air from rising to ceiling.

Insulate pipes that carry hot water. Wrap old towels around them. Be sure to wrap cold water pipes also to stop condensation that can cause mold.

Replace filters on your forced air heating system every month during heating season. For help with changing filters, see chapter on how to change filters.

The Hardware Store: HIS Turf.
Now it's YOURS!

Like we've said before, YOUR new best friend is the man who works in the local hardware store. YOUR pal, just plain Pete. Why? Because HE knows almost every item of the hundreds, maybe thousands of items he has in stock, and when things break, wear out, what YOU need to fix them.

"BUT THE HARDWARE STORE IS A MAN'S WORLD"

NOT IS…WAS.

Now it's YOUR turf. Show him how much you need him, and he (smart business-man that he is) will be flattered, and lucky you, helpful. Women like us do not question his knowledge. And that's good for his ego and his bottom line.

Bring in the blown light bulb and he will guide you to the right one for that specific antique lamp, or your high-intensity convection oven.

And while you're there, you can get advice about your toast-r-oven that bakes but won't top brown, etc. HE could never figure out why. PETE CAN AND DOES.

I have a love for plastic storage containers in all shapes and sizes, and here's where Pete shines with information on all the newest bowls, bins and everything in between. Where could YOU find metal slide out shelves that you nail into your pantry which, bless them, hold dozens of canned soups and baking supplies tidily? Pete knows, and he will even show you how to install them.

The man in your house may have known how to sharpen knives but his organiza-tion skills were probably less than top drawer. Again, once you've established a one-to one relationship with your neighborhood hardware store professional, you'll appreciate having help around the corner.

Note: If you're not lucky enough to have a "Pete", check out the local Home Depot or Lowe's. Or ask a friend for a recommendation. Trust us, this man can and will be a life saver.

A Feel Good Page

Like we've been telling you.

Like you've been realizing more and more each day that...

YES...

YOU can do

what HE used to do.

Ready to learn more? Let's go.....

The Pilot Light:
How to Light it When You're Flying Solo

This is a sensitive subject...ESPECIALLY If HE was the one that poked his head into the oven, or fiddled with the pilot light on the gas stove or the one on the water heater. This is definitely a NO NO.

No matter how adept HE was at fixing, NO ONE, MALE, OR FEMALE, SHOULD TAMPER WITH ANYTHING THAT INVOLVES GAS. That goes for gas water heaters. Gas ovens. Gas stoves. Gas dryers. Gas Lamps. Gas anything.

If the pilot light is not working, IMMEDIATELY call your local gas company, and report the problem. They will tell you if YOU need to abandon ship until they arrive. They will also give you any instructions to follow until they get there.

And this goes for a gas jet on your stove top that sputters, lights for a few seconds and then extinguishes. Something's wrong that could endanger your life and others. Better to be safe than sorry.

Having gone through two french fry fires and my best friends' family room fire, I speak from experience. Call for help immediately, and evacuate family, pets, and yourself.

Moving Furniture Inside and Out
Without Needing a Chiropractic Adjustment

Hello Dolly. Remember the last time you moved, and those big brawny guys flexed their biceps while you wished you were either 20 years younger or had done those arm push-ups religiously?

Now YOU're on your own, and moving furniture is not on your agenda. But somebody's gotta do it and that somebody could be YOU.

Invest in a three month membership in the fitness club? Probably not.

Better still, invest in one of those mover's dollys…those hand trucks you can pick up (literally) at Home Depot. Harder to find, but worth the effort are the ones your local mover, UPS, FED EX, and/or furniture store uses. These are also useful for moving outdoor furniture from inside to outside without breaking your back figuratively and literally.

I've also found them incredibly useful for lugging books from the apartment to the car to the donation bin at the local library. And I met a very attractive and chivalrous teacher who came to my aid unloading the trunk of my car. (That's another story).

Consider also adding rollers to tables and chairs and sofas (beds usually come with built-in casters that slide easily over carpets and wood floors). So when YOU decide to move things around or out, you can do it easily.

Yes, we said YOU.

HELPS YOU DO WHAT HE USED TO DO **67**

Insects and Other Pests:
Don't Get Bugged

Embarrassing as it may sound, despite being cleaning fanatics, bugs happen. Spiders, bed bugs, fleas and the whole gang can find happiness in YOUR abode. HIS job was getting rid of the bad guys.

Now that HIS job is YOUR job, check out what your local hardware store or home improvement center carries. It's wise to keep de-buggers on hand for emergency situations. Spring seems to be their (ants especially) breeding time, and they go into high gear come summer.

Here are some suggestions from our very savvy person at the local hardware store:

Glue traps work well for bugs and mice. Unfortunately, the next step after you catch the culprit may not be to your liking. GET A NEIGHBOR, THE SUPER, OR A VERY GOOD FRIEND TO HELP.

Keep ant traps away from pets for very obvious reasons. If you live in a newly built apartment building, watch out for ant colonies and cockroaches. And if you have groceries delivered, discard boxes and bags immediately. Cockroaches love to hang out in them.

As for the termites and major menaces that sprays couldn't handle, HE handed them off to the exterminating service. On the surface that seems a wise decision.

ON THE SURFACE.

Before you send for and spend for a bonafide exterminator, read this bonafide story of what can go wrong:

My husband was the chief in charge of getting those men in the unmarked trucks to come to our house. For fifteen years Joe "visited", poking around and sharing a cup of "Joe" with my husband before and after he spritzed the magic spray. Nice guy. From a reputable company.

Fast forward 15 years, husband gone, widow puts house up for sale, prospective buyer has house checked out. Inspector finds massive termite damage on staircase leading to cellar, other damage along cellar wall. Sale of house falls through.

Now what? First, I fired the existing company, and when they insisted we had a contract, I pointed out what happened with the house sale.

Next, I interviewed several exterminating companies. Which you should do.

In addition, get references. Check references. Then, have that company come to the house or apartment and detail what they plan to do.

For instance, the company I chose demonstrated why I had termites and termite damage. It appears that the holes bored outside by Company X for injecting the magic potions were never bored deep enough. So, for 15 years, wood inside became the breeding ground for hungry termites. Result: a staircase to the basement held up by a thread, and some fat and happy termites.

Lesson Learned!!!! Get competitive quotes. Check references.

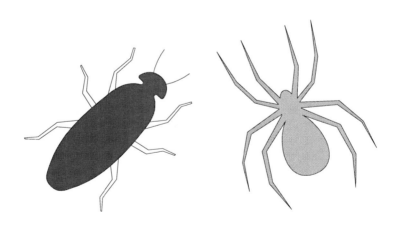

Not to be Overlooked:
Mold Detection

Mold can play havoc with your possessions and your health. HE may not have been up to speed with this bad guy. But YOU should be...especially if you live in an old house or aging apartment.

Mold menaces your belongings, your lungs, your general well-being. If you have any suspicion that you might have a mold problem: a cough, a lingering cold, sudden fatigue, lack of energy, call for help. ASAP. Get someone in to check the air quality, signs of mold, and advice on how to get rid of mold and mold damage.

Equally important, get yourself to a doctor for a top to bottom check-up. Quite frankly, your life may be at risk. Don't take chances. Get professionals to check out your home and you. Today!

Turning Off the Outside Water in Fall; Turning it Back on in Spring

First, locate the outside faucet and pipe that delivers water from inside. Now, locate pipe inside — probably in basement — that delivers water outside. Mine has a red handle. Shut off water by tightening handle. Now go outside and open faucet slightly, allowing air to remain in pipe to keep it from freezing. You are now set for winter.

> **Note:** Don't forget to disconnect hose and roll up and store in the garage or basement. Otherwise you will be buying new hoses every year.

In Spring, turn on water by loosening handle on the same pipe in your basement. Attach hose to outside faucet and test to see if water is flowing freely through pipe.

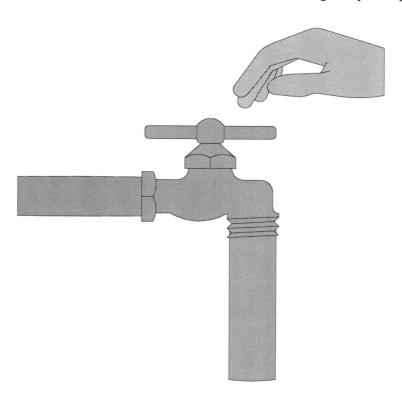

Screens to Storms and Vice Versa

Most screens slide on and off easily. And when spring comes, HE was the one to haul them up from the basement and place them in their usual "nests". Easy. Yes. In winter, he would reverse the process, undo them and return them to the basement.

When it came to be MY duty, I stepped up to the plate and thought, "Piece of cake". Yes, it was easy to lift them up, stack them, and put them in the basement.

EXCEPT FOR ONE MAJOR ERROR: WHEN I PUT THEM AWAY IN FALL, I OVERLOOKED THE MARKINGS HE HAD PUT ON EACH, I.E. A GOES ON WINDOW A, B ON B, AND SO FORTH.

Spring came, and after spending hours trying to match screens to windows and doors and finally realizing those markings on the frames were specific instructions, I broke the code.

Lesson here: mark each and every screen in ink designating where it should go to each and every window and door. EASY, isn't it?

Cleaning Up and Clearing Out

Yeah, we know what can happen. HE promised to clean out the attic, clear out the storage space, empty the catch-all closet, but somehow never got around to it. It wasn't HIS top priority.

Now the ball is in your court, along with the back copies of National Geographics, HIS College Yearbooks, clothes, rolled up carpeting, etc. Here's how to avoid a melt-down:

Assess what is worth keeping and what can be tossed. Be ruthless. Old hand-me-downs like parkas and pants that have been there for 10 years are O U T. HIS heavy luggage, though charming to look at, is also a bye-bye.

Make a list of what you want to keep, what can be donated, and what belongs in the throw-out bin or dumpster.

Set aside "the keepers".

Take a break.

Another Feel Good Page

Like we've been telling you.

Like you've been realizing more and more each day that....

YES! YOU can do what HE did on your own. Now don't you feel better?

YES!

Onward and Upward
More Cleaning Up and Clearing Out

Now, repeat the same steps we talked about earlier—cleaning up and clearing out. This time, be even more ruthless. You will be surprised at how much lighter and better YOU feel.

Note: Check sources for donating at end of this chapter.

Sources for Donating, Giving, etc.

Clothing & Furniture: Search on the internet or yellow pages for locations of:

Local Salvation Army Donation Center

Local Goodwill Donation Center

Big Brother/Big Sister

American Cancer Society

Specific causes you are involved with, interested in

Most will pick up especially if it involves furniture, large donations

Magazines, Books: Check with local schools, colleges and hospitals. They will give you details for donating

Note: Don't forget to get stamped receipts for reporting any and all donations on your income tax.

Automobile: The internet can help you find sources to donate cars and get income tax deductions or cash. Google it.

Skis, Sports Equipment, Exercise Equipment: Again, these donations can be included in your income tax deductions for charity reports.

You could also ask your kids, relatives, friends, neighbors, if they have need for/ want any of what's there, i.e. dishes, utensils, bric-a-brac. If they say no, continue with the task at hand, get a dumpster, and trash them.

NOW, let the fresh air in, and a fresh start begin.

The Barbecue
(A Man's Domain...Until NOW!)

One of the last bastions of male machismo is the barbecue. Over it, HE reigns supreme.

Now comes your turn to grill, roast, kebob and anything in between.

Rather than being intimidated by it, make it YOUR friend. Every barbecue, gas or charcoal, comes with a handbook which clearly spells out the actual cooking process, i.e. recipe, preparation, cooking time, etc. Just like cooking on the inside oven. Let's track it step by step, starting with a charcoal fire, which has been revered by outdoor cooking aficionados since cavemen and women days.

Rule #1, whether you use a charcoal grill or a gas grill, is to allow enough time for the grill to be hot, with a charcoal grill 25 to 30 minutes (coals should have a light coating of light ash), with a gas grill 10 to 15 minutes. Now for the specifics.

The Charcoal Grill

Prepare the fire. Remove cooking grate (where you put food you will be cooking). Add 12-14 pieces of charcoal/charcoal briquettes to kettle/cooker. Squirt charcoal lighter fluid on charcoal, light, and when embers begin to turn red, replace cooking grate with food you are going to cook, cover kettle/cooker and cook for time specified in cook book. Make sure you open vent on cooking hood if yours has one.

> **Tip:** Don't forget to clean cooking rack and remove embers before or after using barbecue.

> **Tip:** Cleaning the grill is easy when you soak overnight. Fill large pan big enough to hold entire grill grate with warm water. Add Spic 'n Span, let sit overnight, rinse and put back on barbecue.

The Gas Grill

Gas grills use gas. Specifically propane gas. So you must be sure you either have a propane tank or a gas line attached to your grill. Empty propane tanks can be taken to local gas station to exchange for filled ones. Hardware stores carry propane, too.

> **Tip:** Most gas grills do not have readings on the side to tell you when you will be out of propane. Err on the safe side and lift up tank every 6 weeks to guess how much is left. Better yet, keep a spare tank on hand.

Open switch to ignite propane. Follow specific instructions in recipe. Still unsure: for meats and poultry use an instant read thermometer. Or use sharp knife to cut into the meat or poultry to test "doneness".

Look at you! You're a bonafide Outdoor Chef!

> **Tip:** Same cleaning tip applies here. See above.

Digging, Mulching, Mowing—
More Man-ual Labor

If you don't live in a house, you can skip this chapter, relax and perhaps stir up something delicious in the kitchen.

If YOU do have a garden, a small dear-to-your-heart piece of land, read on. Especially if HE was the extra pair of hands to grow, stow, and mow.

Begin with checking to see what garden tools YOU have on hand. Briefly, you need the following:

A **hoe** and/or a pitchfork to dig up clumps of soil and use for seeds and/or plants

A **lightweight rake** usually with bamboo "fingers" for raking leaves

A heavier **fork rake** for aerating soil, spreading mulch, smoothing out and cleaning up beds

A **pruner** to cut and groom plants and small shrubs

A **bulb planter** if you are into bulbs

A **trowel**, a small hand shovel

Gardening gloves, good heavy ones, cheapie **knee pads**, an oversize **hat** to protect against the sun

And don't forget the **SUN BLOCK** fair lady

Note: You may want to chuck some of these if they're man-size tools, too heavy and burdensome. Before you do, give them a work-out to check what to keep and what to get rid of. Most definitely, YOU need to buy gloves to fit your hands.

Besides the usual hardware and gardening stores close to where you live, big chains like Lowe's and Home Depot are excellent sources of gardening tools, plants and information.

How-to books? Check Amazon.com or the local hardware and/or gardening stores. Don't take on more than you can handle, especially if you're a neophyte.

A window sill herb garden can be as enlightening and fulfilling as a small patch of earth outside your front door.

But start small. Gardening should be a labor of love, not simply labor. Try a tomato "tree" in a pot, or force bulbs for winter displays. They all come with easy to follow directions.

> **Tip:** Check the Sources for Gardening Tools for Women at the end of this chapter and the How-To Booklets at the local hardware store, gardening store or home improvement center.

As for tougher jobs like mowing the lawn, heavy weeding, cutting back overgrowth, get HELP. Most men do this once or maybe twice then move onto TV and reading the paper after they call a local landscaper to take over the heavy duty jobs.

YOU can do likewise. Have fun!

Sources for Gardening Tools for Women

Beyond the local gardening center and home improvement center, there are many choices for gardening tools for women that can be found on-line.

Garden, Artisans: Offers high quality gardening tools, many ergonomically correct for women

DIY Woman: Offers good quality gardening tools for woman with grips made for a woman's smaller hands. Check out their website at: www.DIYWoman.com

Target: Check on line site www.target.com . Or at store near where you live. Target offers a variety of different sets from the basics to ones made of high quality stainless steel, along with light and heavy duty gardening gloves and boots, even a knee rest to protect your knees while tending to your plants.

The following offer full-size digging tools designed by and for women:

Victorian Postman Limited

Ames

Spear & Jackson

www.Sears.com

All are lighter in weight, sometimes with fiberglass handles instead of wood.

The Car:
Beyond Putting the Key in and Starting it

First, some essential reading: The Driver's Manual. You're never ever going to read it end to end. But YOU should open it and mark some important pages. For example, the service schedule. Yes, it does need to be serviced on a regular basis based on mileage accrued. Your manual will give you the specifics.

It's especially important to have the oil checked and changed at regular intervals, noted in the manual and in another chapter in this book. This simple task can save you unexpected, and what could be very expensive, aggravation.

If you're taking over HIS car, beyond re-registration, insurance and other details described in later chapters, you need to be familiar with HIS particular model. Again, and this is important, you should refer to the driver's manual. Important, too, is having a full service check-out before you take over ownership. The adage Better Safe than Sorry makes sense.

Other sections to make note of: adjusting seats and head rests. Adjusting rear and side view mirrors. All vital to protecting you against major accidents and minor mishaps. HE was probably a big help here. But now YOU are in the driver's seat, for better or for worse.

The manual will also remind you what grade of gas to use. The manual will show and tell you what the icons on your dashboard/cockpit mean. Which light beams to use when and where. How to use Cruise Control. How to child-proof the car. How the heating system and AC works.

UH-OH: HE went bye-bye. So did the car manual. Go on line to contact manufacturer for a replacement. Often, too, used car dealers carry them.

Other Necessary Reading

Another chapter to check out: warning lights. Most of us wait until the warning light pops on to figure out what to do next. Or worse yet, panic. A better scenario is to glance over that section in your manual so you have some knowledge of what COULD happen. A quick review of the dashboard and which indicators mean what function is mal-functioning is a necessity before driving HIS car. And YOURS.

Often, the warning light will give you time to get to a service station to check out what's wrong. What's important is to heed the warning. Don't ignore it. Remember there's no Mr. Fix-it around to fix it.

One other reminder: check out the manual for advice about transporting children safely. YOU'll feel better knowing you're buckling up correctly. And so will they.

IMPORTANT: DON'T read the manual while driving. Stop, read, react. IF A WARNING LAMP TURNS ON, RESPECT IT.

And unless you have an ear piece, DO NOT DRIVE AND TALK ON YOUR CELL. DO NOT DRIVE AND TEXT MESSAGE. ABSOLUTELY POSITIVELY DO NOT.

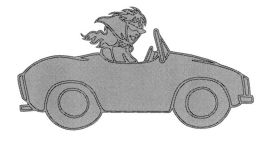

How to Turn Pumping Your Own Gas into an Uplifting Experience

This sounds like a dumb idea at first glance. WRONG. Full service stations work on the premise that lots of women want full service. And are willing to PAY FULL PRICE for this service. Besides, there was usually a man around to do the fill-ups.

NOT ANYMORE.

The time has come to pump YOUR own gas. Let's first discuss the advantages: number one, it saves you time. No waiting for an attendant. No waiting for a receipt.

Number two, it saves you money. No ten cents or more a gallon for service rather than self-service. A year's worth could save you hundreds of dollars. And number three, YOU are in control of the situation. Nice feeling, eh?

Here's how you do it: Go to tanks in aisles marked "Self-Service". Make sure you are parked on the correct side of the tanks where you can easily reach your gas tank, and that the engine is turned off. Open hatch to gas tank, unscrew cap. Now follow instructions on front panel of gas tanks. They will take you through paying by credit card, or cash, choosing grade you want, and getting the go ahead to fill your tank. Press correct buttons, and begin to fill tank. As long as you press down on hose, gas will flow into tank.

You decide how much gas you want to buy, or fill tank completely. Machine will then print out receipt if you ask for one. Close and tighten tank cap, and close hatch.

Tip: The driver's manual will tell you what grade gas to use. You'll save more money using the correct grade for your particular model car.

Putting Air in Tires: How do YOU do it?

First, if you're like many women, you have to overcome your fear of failure. YOU CAN DO IT. So go for it.

Next, you have to convince yourself that no way will you risk life nor limb doing this. Count on some inexplicable law of physics to prevent a serious miss-step or mishap.

Important: STOP AND READ THE DRIVER'S MANUAL. This gives pre-scribed amount of air pressure needed for your specific model of car. Now park close to the air pump and unwind the hose, unscrew the cap on the tire, extend the hose getting as close as you can to the tire. Fill the tire following the guidelines in the manual. Close the cap, re-wind the hose, and you're on your way.

This is one of the most satisfying lessons I learned being on my own. And starting today, YOU are on your way to being in control on your own.

> **Tip:** If your car is older and the manual has been lost or bought used without the manual, you will find amount of air pressure needed on the door. The internet is also an excellent source of this type of information.

Also, this is a good time to mention rotating tires. For sure HE was the car maven, and attended to having YOUR car serviced as well as HIS own. Now you're the one who has to make sure the service people rotate the tires, change the oil, check the windshield wipers, and keep your car in tip top condition. And don't forget to make sure your tires are good for winter travel as well as during the rest of the year.

> **Tip:** Keeping track of service records is easier when you enter time and date each time you have your car serviced. Keep records handy in the glove compartment. (See Chapter on Glove Compartment.)

Breakdowns, Flats and Other Mishaps

Just when YOU thought life was running on a fairly smooth path, bingo, you get a flat. Panic? No. You've got roadside service, and they'll be there in no time. Right? If you're lucky, they will be. If you're way out in the "boonies", you're going to have to wait.

Before we go any further, please make note of the following:

Very important to keep the telephone number of roadside service in your car, and accessible in your glove compartment. Equally important is to keep an extra card in your wallet just in case you've forgotten that it's in the glove compartment. And lady in distress — keep the telephone number noted on your cell phone directory. Chances are you'll remember one out of three.

Next, give them accurate information of where you are, i.e. exit number, street, road, any other signs that would be helpful. Give them your cell number. Make of car, license plate, any other information that can help them get to you pronto.

AND LOCK YOUR CAR!

Important: If HE handled the insurance, roadside service, etc., make sure everything is paid for and up to date. We've covered this and other necessities in later chapters. When you're stuck on a deserted country road is no time to ask yourself "Do I have roadside service?"

Generally, roadside will change tire, or give you a "donut" to carry you temporarily.

    Tip: Again, be cautious. Ask for I.D., proof that THEY are legitimate. And keep your cell phone ON.

Found:
The Dark, Mysterious, Puzzling Glove Compartment...in HIS and YOUR Car

When was the last time YOU opened the glove department in your car? Or his?

Now's the time to check it out. Important to remember is the fact that besides stowing sun tan lotion and extra lipsticks, this is where YOU should keep your car registration, your insurance cards and information, and your roadside assistance card and information. Equally important is to keep these cards up to date. And the insurance premiums paid.

If you have ever had a flat tire, or other mishap, you realize how important it is to have everything in one place, ready, willing and able to get you out of a jam and up and running again.

I also keep a note pad and pen for marking down directions, vital phone numbers like the baby sitter, doctor, neighbor, my brother's care giver. And the nice man at the local gas station. Just in case.

Next, in order of importance, a flashlight. Someone gifted me with a small one that comes with extra batteries, and it has been a godsend in an emergency situation. I consider it a safety measure as well, particularly if you get stuck on a rainy night halfway from home. This, and my cell phone give me great comfort at this time of my life.

IMPORTANT TO NOTE HERE: Make sure to check the batteries in the flashlight periodically. And re-charge the cell phone when you can. Better now than later. Better safe, than sorry. We can't emphasize that too many times.

Next, the driver's manual with more information than you need in a lifetime. Mine is too fat to fit in the glove compartment so I keep the necessary pages/books here, and the remainder in the trunk of my car.

Of lesser importance: It's handy to have a cotton rag to help clean windshield and side windows in bad weather.

Now, you can tuck in the lipsticks, sun tan lotions, and chewing gum, if there's room.

P.S. You might consider putting your EZ Pass in the glove compartment as well…for security reasons. Because you CAN lock your glove compartment.

The Car Trunk: A Good Hiding Place

HE probably stowed everything in the trunk: his golf clubs, your tennis racket, the cooler, the recyclables for the pick up drive, kids parkas, friends T-shirts, and so on.

We mention this because at this time of your life YOU don't need further clutter. Part of taking stock of what you should keep and what you should toss is discussed in chapters ON GETTING ORGANIZED and CLEANING UP AND CLEARING OUT.

Once you've pared down the contents of the car trunk, consider what should be kept there: a snow shovel and an extra can of de-icer for winter emergency, an old blanket which can come in handy if you get stuck on a slippery road, along with extra rags to clean windshields, headlights, etc. Also, the spare tire or doughnut. No, you're not going to attempt to change a flat. That's what Roadside Service is all about. And don't forget the rest of the Service Manual. Today, they're as bulky and weighty as the World Atlas. Keep important pages in the Glove Compartment. (SEE SECTION ON GLOVE COMPARTMENT) The rest in your trunk. Not essential, but not a bad idea: an extra cooler that you can use when you do a big shop and need to keep perishables cold.

Get Regular Check-Ups — for Your Car and His

Now that the keys are in your pocket, YOU have to make sure to get the car inspected, renew the insurance, and have it serviced on regular occasions, the things HE probably did for you. Important to keep in mind are the following:

The manual, specific section on service, will tell you how often YOU need to have the oil changed, rotate the tires, and in winter if you live where snow and ice happen, make sure your tires are prepped for bad weather. If they need snow tires, BUY THEM. It's your life. You're on your own now.

And DON'T delay check-ups on a regular basis.

> **Note:** If your car is still under factory warranty, you are in luck. Regular check-ups are part of the deal. If your warranty period is nearing its end, check with the dealer to see if you can extend it.

Make a list of what needs to be addressed like windshield wipers, a funny light that comes on and you can't figure out what it means. A buzz that happens when you turn on the radio. Yes, you can check the manual, but sad to admit, it is written in MAN TALK. It's OK to admit you're not a born mechanic. And trust us, you will get help.

Truth be told, most women NEVER EVER read the car manual. OF COURSE HE DID. But what HE did and what YOU have to do is totally different. I know we've covered this in another chapter, but it's worth repeating.

At least read the section that enlightens you to what the dashboard icons mean. AND FOLLOW THE INSTRUCTIONS.

> **Tip:** Should your car need repairs, make sure to get several estimates. Ninety-nine out of 100 women are not car mechanics and have no — sorry to admit — knowledge of costs of repairs and parts. A male friend recommended taking him long for the appraisal. I think I saved half!!

Once you've got the car thing under your belt, make a date to have a check-up for yourself.

Checking the Oil Level:
Now it's a Job for a Woman

HE knew how to check the oil level. Do YOU?

First, make sure you check out the car manual to see what those signals that seem to pop up on the instrument panel...just when you don't expect them...mean. If the one that says check oil level shows, go to the nearest gas station, and ask them to show you where the oil stick is. CLUE: IT'S UNDER THE HOOD. Next, lift out oil stick, wipe it with a cloth or paper towel (available at the pump), dip it into the opening, and see how high or low your oil level is. These sticks usually have markings on them to show levels of oil.

Low level? Have the attendant do it or do it yourself. Add a quart or two as needed. Tighten cap, and you're done.

If you have oil changed at your regular service check-ins, they will paste sticker with date, mileage and place it on windshield on driver's side to remind you of next service call and/or next oil change. Some service stations place reminder sticker on inside door panel on driver's side.

Mission accomplished.

NOTE: FAILING TO CHANGE OIL AT REGULAR INTERVALS CAN BE A VERY EXPENSIVE MISTAKE. Check the oil level periodically or have the service people do it when you have your regular check-up.

Outfitting the Car for Bad Weather

Ice and snow. Drifts and stalled cars. Temperatures in the low digits. You shiver just thinking of those bad guys.

Note: If you live where the sun shines 24/7, 365 days a year, you can skip this chapter.

BUT if you're faced with ugly weather three or four months of the year, if not more, take note of the following advice:

Now that you're on your own, YOU need to be prepared. Here's what you need:

Windshield wipers that are new and working properly

De-icer for frozen locks and frozen windows

Ice scraper and **snow brush**

A shovel —a good one — and if you can find one, a telescoping one that can fit in your trunk

A traction mat (sold on line and in automotive supply stores) that will get you out of snow, ice and mud. They go under one of the drive wheels to give your car the traction it needs to get going.

A cell phone with your roadside assistance number locked in

Other useful cold weather information:

Let car warm up before you take off in cold weather. Even though water temperature may show that the car is warming up, the oil inside the engine takes longer. The reason: oil is denser than water. Which means you may have to wait 10 minutes longer before driving. Same goes for transmission and shock absorbers. Be patient on cold days.

Washing Your Car
HE DID IT—Sometimes

Have you checked the prices at the drive-though car wash recently?

Outrageous! I could make a down payment on a new Honda for what my local guy charges. So I bit the bullet and decided that I was going to try and wash my own car.

First I tried convincing one of my kids home from college to do it. The pay wasn't "agreeable". We (read He) decided we'd flip a coin.

Unfortunately, I didn't win the toss up.

However, I did realize I could do it! Better still, I found that I actually enjoy washing my car. What used to be HIS or Their job is now mine. And once I got the hang of it, I actually pride myself on a job well done.

My way: A bucket of soapy water or a solution specially made for washing cars
    An over-size sponge
    Big, used towels and/or chamois
    A garden hose or a very, very large bucket or both

Step 1. Hose or douse car down with water from big bucket

Step 2. Apply soapy water or special car washing solution to car, preferably starting with cleaner areas, i.e. windows, windshield, headlights and back lights, then bumpers, frame of car, ending with tires and hubs. Tires and hubs generally need 2 or 3 passes as they get the grease. Again, there are special cleaners for these parts if you're really into being the top car washer on your block.

Step 3. Run hose over entire car. Again you can use buckets of water, but this takes longer. Dry with chamois or big towels.

Step 4. Admire.

Washing the windows? No way. Solution: Pay somebody.

Getting Organized:
YOUR Way vs. HIS Way

Most of us are not as organized as we'd like to think we are. HE had a system, not a perfect one, but it was a system. What about YOU?

For instance, where do YOU keep the Use and Care books for your Toast-r-Oven? The service contract for your washing machine? The key to the safety deposit box? The deeds, bank statements?

Yes, they're there somewhere. Out there. Now's the time to determine what's important to have close at hand in case of an emergency, and what can go in a file, or desk drawer or safety deposit box.

Let's start with keys.

Lost and Found:
Keys to the House, Car, Safety Deposit Box, etc.
a.k.a. I never met a key I didn't like.

I get anxious just reading the title to this chapter. And YOU probably do, too.

Even if you consider yourself buttoned up, well organized, on top of it, you have found yourself in a panic state looking for the keys to the basement closet, the extra set for the car, his car, and so forth.

Now's the time to tally up what to keep, what to toss, and what to put in a safe, easily accessible place. Not the sugar bowl. But a safe, accessible place.

Let's start with the obvious: the keys to the house. ASSIGN A DRAWER in your kitchen or desk. Clear out that drawer so you have space for the keys.

> **Note:** Your mom's favorite fudge recipe, your first valentine, etc. have got to go.

VERY OBVIOUS BUT ALSO VERY IMPORTANT: MARK THE KEYS with tags. Sounds duhhhhh, but if you have ever searched for keys in the dead of night, you will appreciate having done this.

NEXT, and equally important, throw out the keys to the old apartment, keys you can't figure out where they belong, keys that are bent. The old adage, "when in doubt, throw it out" fits here.

Along with the keys to the house, the extra set of keys to the car should be kept here. Marked.

> **Note:** An alternative suggestion is discussed in chapter on safekeeping important papers.

The mail box key, with a duplicate, is also kept here. Again, clearly marked. I also keep an extra mail box key for my condo neighbor who cheerfully takes in my mail and packages when I'm away.

Don't forget the safety deposit key. You may not think so, but it is a good idea to invest in a safety deposit box for important papers, stock certificates, jewelry and anything you wouldn't want to risk being stolen or misplaced. Or worse still, being destroyed in a fire.

I keep my safety deposit keys (our bank gives you two) in this same drawer along with the other keys. My safety deposit keys come in an envelope. I've noted the box number on the outside, which is necessary for getting into the vault in my bank.

> **Note:** For more safekeeping information, see chapter on safety deposit box.

Any additional keys, back door to your house or apartment, entry door of apartment building, office keys, etc. belong in this drawer. Clearly marked. I can't emphasize this enough.

> **Important P.S.** Throughout the years of moving and traveling, I've amassed a collection of keys. All of which have been put in the throw out pile, hesitantly, for "just in case". Well, now's the time to get rid of them. So go for it. Do it!

Now don't you feel much lighter?

Service Providers:
Make a List, and Check it Twice

Here's where YOU come into your own. You are slowly but surely getting a handle on things. How to fix a toilet. How to change a filter. How to flip a mattress. The ins and outs of car maintenance.

One step at a time.

Which brings us to a discussion of getting organized.

In our house, my husband kept track of bills to be paid, services to be ordered, clean ups and clean outs.

HE also kept a note pad in his desk with the names of all the service providers from the guy who plowed our driveway in winter to the people who delivered the daily newspaper. Unfortunately, the note pad organizational method gave way to pieces of paper stuck in drawers in the kitchen, inside the telephone directory, in his agenda and appointment book.

Starting over means really starting over.

Buy a notebook and mark it: IMPORTANT PHONE NUMBERS!!!!

Make sure it's an alphabetized notebook or one with tabs so you can indicate the correct phone number for the plumber, etc.

Now check any numbers HE used to be sure they are still in business. If so, and you are happy with their service, note in the notebook, with a tab that says Plumbers.

Follow this same procedure with any other numbers of household services you find, always checking them out before entering them in YOUR book.

Once you've finished this task, put your book in a readily accessible place: next to your phone in the kitchen, on your bedside table. Ready, willing and able to come to your aid night and day.

Just in case, BACK-UP YOUR list of service providers on your computer.

Which brings us to suggesting backing up this very important list, critical to your everyday happiness. Back up names, addresses, phone numbers and e-mails for all your service providers by inputting them into your computer, saving the list, and bookmarking it: SERVICE PROVIDERS.

And keep it up to date. You may even want to add comments after you use these service people, i.e. ask for Joe, pay cash and get a discount, etc.

Aren't YOU the organized one!

> **Note:** If you don't have a computer, make a copy of this list and keep it where it's easily accessible. In that desk drawer that you've delegated to safekeeping.

Safekeeping:
Use & Care Of Books, Service Contracts, etc.

You might not consider a warranty/use and care booklet valuable, but when the thermostat breaks down and you haven't a clue of what to do, you'll wish you knew where the warranty booklet was hiding. MR. Fix-it doesn't live here any more, and YOU've got to do the fix-its. YOU wish you had a special place for them. And they were all in one place.

If you have the space, put all the warranty books in one place, in a kitchen drawer. OR A DESK DRAWER. Ollie keeps hers in a file cabinet in the small office off her kitchen. That way, she has easy access should a problem arise.

Here's where YOU should also keep information about ordering spare parts. They're usually noted on a separate sheet that comes with your appliance.

> **Note:** It's a good idea to check out your collection of booklets, guarantee cards, and toss the ones that are no longer valid. Like the one for the iron you bought 10 years ago which is now long gone.

As you buy new appliances, fill out the warranty cards and mail them in. HE probably did. YOU should, too. Because when something goes wrong, they'll fix it. Guaranteed.

Case in Point: Marilyn M, newly on-her-own, discovered one night that her automatic garage door had a mind of its own. It refused to stay closed. She found the warranty card and the phone number of the company located somewhere out West. Luckily, a helpful customer service person walked her through how to correct the problem. Step by step. Now YOU understand why it's important to have a place for those warranty books, service contracts, and emergency phone numbers.

Safekeeping:
Documents, Deeds and Done Deals

Admittedly, in our home, HE was in charge of safekeeping the valuables and the paperwork: the wills, the income tax reports, the closing documents, the bank accounts, the titles to the car, the stock brokerage accounts, the things we all dread to do and probably never did.

The closest I ever came to storing valued papers was buying an expandable file. And that disappeared somewhere in one of the many moves I've made over the years.

What's more scary, my husband handled the tax reports, the deeds, the surveys, closing documents on property we owned, paid bills, did all the financial stuff and HE put them in one deep, dark drawer in his desk. Luckily, for me, a complete financial dummy, these valuable documents were easy to find.

Most of us aren't that lucky. So let's get a handle on it. First, buy an expandable file. A good sturdy one. Or delegate several drawers of a file cabinet to storing home documents. and if you've outgrown the file cabinet, either get another or designate part of a closet to keeping records. Milk crates can work here. With files labelled and properly organized.

Next, make sure to label the files accordingly, i.e. tax bills, income tax reports, insurance payments, mortgage payments, credit car payments, utility payments, title to the car, etc.

Note: The law requires saving income tax reports for 7 years. And it's wise to keep business and personal financial documents like receipts for up to 10 years in case you get audited. Unless your lawyer or accountant insists that you hold onto these records longer than prescribed by law, be strong and toss them.

One caveat here: If you are not sure what to keep and what to toss, KEEP for the time being. Once you get a better feel for what you're doing, you can periodically review and decide then what to keep and what to toss.

I also have a separate file cabinet devoted to stock reports, monthly reports from bank and brokerage houses; stock certificates are kept in my safety deposit box.

An aside here: Many of us pay our bills online. If so, print out information and put a copy of each in your designated file. That way, you can keep track of expenditures and get a fix on how to budget monies.

If all else fails, get a financial advisor to set up a system, and follow it. Accountants can also be helpful here.

Note: For help on finding and choosing a financial advisor, see chapter on Financial Advisors

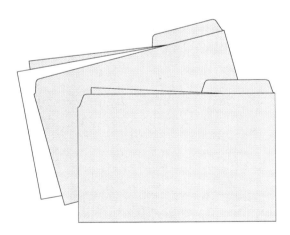

Managing Your Own Finances vs. Getting Outside Help

You may decide YOU want to manage your own finances. Be aware that this requires hours of research and learning. If YOU decide to do this, you need to recognize that it is incredibly time consuming, particularly if you're at the bottom of the learning curve. And BE SURE you have the discipline to stay the course, to think rationally rather than emotionally. Do-it-yourself investors often allow their emotions to dictate their investment decisions.

For many amateur investors, inflation is a risk that is often overlooked. It may FEEL comfortable keeping your investments in a CD. But generally they don't keep pace with inflation; YOU often run the risk of asset deterioration over time.

If your financial needs are simple, straight forward, and you're not risking the family fortune, you probably can fold this into your accountant's or lawyer's responsibility.

If they're more complex, we suggest you consult an outside expert. Someone beyond the accountant who did yours and HIS taxes. Someone besides your lawyer and/or accountant who advises you on money matters.

Enter the financial advisor.

They come in all shapes and sizes. With varying degrees of education, experience, and bedside manner.

How do you go about locating one? Look in the yellow pages? NO. NO. NO. Ask your lawyer. Or your accountant. Ask friends who have used advisors. Contact people who are in the market or deal in financial matters.

If you decide to go the Financial Advisor route, here are some guidelines to keep in mind:

Financial Advisors
First step: Initial interview

Nice news to begin with: in most cases, the first interview is free.

You will get an immediate comfort level or lack of such by sitting down and spending an hour or two with these people. Also, it's wise to choose a financial advisor in your area for face-to-face meetings.

Be prepared. Questions to Ask:

Average account size. Are you a typical client for this advisor?

Risk tendencies. Are they conservative/aggressive enough for your needs and objectives?

Fees and Commissions. How do they get paid?

Favored investment vehicles. Do they prefer individual securities or mutual funds and why?

Existence of liability insurance

How long have they been conducting business in the area?

Availability of references

Any disciplinary actions

They will also explain how they work, i.e. reports, contact on a regular basis, fees. All of this makes sense realizing that most of us are at the bottom of the learning curve.

Be Prepared. Information to bring:

To get the most out of the interview, gather as much information as YOU have, i.e. financial documents, assets and debts. Prioritize your financial needs and goals (retirement, paying off the mortgage, college planning for children and/or grand-children). Providing specific goals and detailed financial information will lead to a higher quality plan.

Next steps:

Once you choose a financial advisor, they will present you with a financial pro-posal. It should be easy to understand with specific details of how and when you will meet your financial goals. The freer you are with information provided, the happier and more successful you will be.

Note: See Sources for books and publications offering financial advice to widows.

Sources for Financial Help
for Widows, Divorcees, Singles

On Your Own: A widow's passage to emotional and financial well being.

By Alexandra Armstrong, Mary R. Donahue, a certified financial planner and a psychologist. Both have lost loved ones, and have written this book with the purpose of easing the journey for others. Recommended for widows, divorcees, and women in a relationship that involves any financial issues.

The Widow's Financial Survival Guide. Handling money matters on your own.

By Nancy Dunnan. Covers a range of financial topics: from the first few weeks, and getting started on your own, to ten things you need to do right away. Plus insights into managing on your own, setting up a new system for bills and credit cards. Written by a financial expert, commentator and magazine columnist.

Worthwhile reading is chapter on common scams and frauds.

The Wall Street Guide to Planning Your Financial Future. By Kenneth Morris, Alan Siegel, and Virginia Morris.

The Survivor Assistance Handbook: A Guide for Financial Transition. By Mark Colglan, CFP, founder of Plan Your Legacy L.L.C.

The ABC's of Widowhood. By Pat Nowak Coping, counselling, and common sense advice for widows.

Seek and You Shall Find
Help with financials is a website away

Check out these websites for help getting started with being on your own:

National Association for Personal Financial Planners. For help with estimating future expenses including medical, figure out when to start collecting Social Security benefits, pensions, etc.

Alliance of Cambridge Advisors

Both of these offer FEE ONLY planning:

Women's Institute for Financial Education

AARP's Widowed Persons Service. For more information and to locate a widowed persons program near you.

Home Security. Part 1:
The Fire Extinguisher. Burglary Alarm. What You Need to Keep Your Home Safe and Secure

The Fire Extinguisher

Whether you live in an apartment or a home, #1 on your list of must haves are fire extinguishers. Not just one stuck into a closet, but several highly visible extinguishers on each and every floor of your house, including the garage, attic, and basement. And more than one in your apartment. Start with one in the kitchen, and add another or two if your apartment or house is more than one level. Or if the bedroom, for instance, is a distance from the kitchen, buy several.

THIS MAY BE SOMETHING HE WAS IN CHARGE OF. BUT NOW YOU'RE IN CHARGE.

FIRE EXTINGUISHERS should be checked out at the hardware store every 6 months to be sure they are in good, running order. And they should be placed where they can be accessible should a fire occur. Not up in the attic or in the back of the closet with your prom dress from high school. One, in the kitchen pantry is where I keep mine after the French-fries-with-an-attitude incident. Another in the 2nd floor linen closet, and a third on garage wall, fourth in the basement.

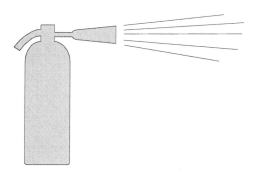

The Burglary Alarm

Equally, if not more important, is a burglary alarm system, the best investment for protection today short of having a large, angry, Police trained dog. Today most houses and apartments come with built-in alarm systems. If yours is pre-installed, make sure the system is up and working. And call the emergency number to be sure they are still in business, and you have a registered account with them.

What a smart lady you are!

Burglary alarms are hooked up to a main monitoring service which you pay for on a continuing basis. It's a good idea to have them check out your key pad, in fact the whole system every few years. Like flashlights, their batteries wear out and need to be replaced periodically.

MAKE SURE YOUR SYSTEM IS HOOKED UP TO THE MAIN MONITORING OFFICE. Sounds dumb, but believe me, this is vital. My office in Greenwich paid for three years of service, and the installer had never hooked it up to the main monitoring headquarters. Even though the president of the company had his office in our building!

If your home or apartment is WITHOUT a built-in system, compare contracts and pricing with several (our financial guru suggests interviewing 3 or 4 companies before you sign a contract). You may also want to call references to check out response times, reliability, pricing, etc.

Home Security. Part 2:
Smoke Alarm

Smoke alarm systems. Often these are folded into the main monitoring system and will signal the local fire station or the central station of a problem at your home. Often, too, the "on your own-ers" choose to install separate smoke sensors throughout the house. Fine, but these need to be serviced on a regular basis to ensure they are functioning 24/7.

Nothing's more irritating than a smoke alarm that goes off when you forgot the lamb chops in the broiler. Mine also has a lovely habit of going off during the night, requiring climbing up and de-fusing it or pulling the covers over my head till morning, then climbing up, de-fusing it, and changing the battery.

Check out YOUR smoke detector to be sure it's working.

Simply press the button on the front. If you hear a loud "beep", that means the batteries and the smoke detector are working. If nothing happens, and there's no "beep", you probably need to change the batteries. Or worse case scenario, you need to buy a new smoke detector. Their life cycle is 7 to 8 years.

We suggest you press the test button each month to be sure it's working properly. And make sure you have a smoke detector on each floor, including the basement. Same goes for condos and apartments, especially in the kitchen.

Changing the batteries. Easy does it:

As you now know, alarms "beep" when their batteries need replacing. Get a step ladder, reach up to the unit and unfasten the unit from the ceiling. Unscrew cover by twisting it to the left and remove batteries. Replace them with new batteries and twist the cover back on. If button doesn't produce a "beep", you may need a new smoke detector.

Sometimes, alarms keep on "beeping" even when you've removed them from the ceiling. Don't be, excuse the pun, alarmed. Trust us, the battery needs replacing.

You'll notice there's a "spring like" piece which holds the battery in place, make sure you press it when you put in the new battery. Replace cap and re-fasten to ceiling.

Tip: Use high quality 9-volt batteries. The old adage you get what you pay for applies here. Store brands and mystery brands do not last as long.

Tip: Have back-up batteries for your alarm system as they wear out faster than you think. Also, note chapter on Back-ups.

Home Security. Part 3:
Carbon Monoxide Detector

Next and probably new to you:

A carbon monoxide detector. That unseen, un-detectable, until it's too late menace can be monitored 24-7 with this essential device. Get one! Or two!

Flashlights. A big, powerful one that can give you lots of light and peace of mind in a sudden black-out. And extra "D" batteries as backup. Another smaller flashlight is a good idea for lighting up smaller spaces. PLUS extra batteries just in case you haven't checked on your emergency safety equipment lately. And candles. Essential when all else fails.

Duct Tape. For emergency fixes

Home Security. Part 4:
In the Garage

Here's an area of YOUR home that is often overlooked in terms of security: the garage. Most garages have windows (usually kept unlocked) and/or a dog door. Both can be entered easily; the intruder then has easy access to YOUR home.

Often, we lock the front door, secure doors to the patio, but leave the door from the garage into the house unlocked. Be aware. Be forewarned.

You'll also want to check out that lock from the back door to inside your house to be sure it's a strong, working lock.

> **Tip:** If you are a new owner of a house or condo with a garage, be sure to re-set the code for the remote garage door opener. And to be extra safe, change all the locks.

Other ways to discourage uninvited guests:

Display Beware of Dog Signs.

And/or invest in a large, loud dog.

Ask a neighbor to park his car in your driveway when you're away.

Put up signs and stickers your security system provides.

MORE ON SECURITY:
Dead Bolt Locks, Motion Detectors, Light/Appliance Timer Switch, and More

Dead Bolt Locks

After her long time boy friend split, Charlene changed the locks on her apartment door. Next, was having the local locksmith put in a dead bolt lock. She also acquired a large Doberman.

If your "nest" doesn't have a built-in alarm system, you should consider one of the three options mentioned above. We've discussed the advantages of a built-in alarm system which provides security 24-7 ONCE YOU ARM THEM. Often, we forget to turn ON the alarm, which makes YOU an easy prey. Whichever you choose, just make sure it's connected, armed, and your dead bolt is locked.

Proof that It Pays to be Fore-Armed: A friend lives in a neighboring development, and has her office in the basement of her condo. Recently, working at home, she found herself facing two large men wielding one even larger knife. They had entered through the front door which was unarmed (security system off) and unlocked in broad daylight. Lucky for the lady, her screams sent them running for cover in the nearest woods.

Moral here: Keep doors locked day and night, night and day. And if you have a security system, keep YOUR security system ON. Remember, YOU are home alone, and you need to feel safe and secure.

Motion Detectors

Amy G who lives on Long Island swears by these. After hosting dinner parties for deer, they loved her rhododendrum and hostas, Amy bought motion detectors and had them mounted on her house, the part that faced her garden. Her Ex thought this was a dopey idea, but along with HIS Exit, went the rabbits, deer and dogs who nibbled on all the delicious greens.

If you're lucky, motion detectors could be the answer to the nocturnal invaders. Once a trespasser crosses the path of a motion detector , BINGO, the light goes on. They might even scare away your EX!

WARNING! DEER ARE SMART, and they can easily figure out motion detectors and continue to eat the shrubbery, the garden. But these are worth a try.

Light/Appliance Timer Switch

Most likely, HE was in charge of this essential home security device. The light/appliance timer that YOU set to go on and off at certain times inside your "nest" while you're away. It can also be used to turn on and off appliances, even the radio. However, as a safety device to discourage uninvited guests, it's a must have.

Note: Make sure you check occasionally to be sure cord is not frayed nor plug worn out. Often a cord hidden under a carpet can fray and burn. (See following page.)

The Step Ladder

What's a step ladder doing in a section marked Security? Right on.

Because step ladders keep our home and family feeling secure. Because they can and do prevent accidents in the home.

For instance, now that HE'S not there to put away the turkey roaster on the top cabinet shelf, your natural instinct is to use a drawer or a chair or the counter top to lift the weighty devil. NO NO NO.

A fold-away step ladder close at hand is the safe and sensible solution. And having one is an absolute necessity. For bigger projects and higher nooks and crannys, you'll probably want to use a major ladder. Again, be sure it is secure when you open it. Better still, get a friend to help.

Frayed Cords & Fire Prevention

We would be remiss not to mention one important fire prevention necessity: cords on electrical appliances. Frayed cords are dangerous and should immediately be replaced.

My recently divorced friend, Mary Ann, had a night light in the large family room which would flip on at assigned hours to discourage burglars and other "drop-ins". Her kids watched TV in that room, danced on the carpet in that room; one night the friction caused the cord to ignite during the wee hours and a three alarm fire resulted. Big time damage.

Luckily, the family and the gerbils were rescued by a hooked up smoke alarm system and a responsive fire department

Back-ups — HE Always had Them. YOU Should, Too.

How frustrating to get set to change the batteries in your flashlight, or the smoke alarm, to find there are NO back up batteries. HE probably kept them in a drawer, kitchen cupboard, or his tool box.

HE also made a habit of replacing them every few months. Like a good son-in-law who has "extras" for the kids' toys.

Beyond batteries, glue sticks, crazy glue, extra pair of heavy duty gloves, clips for fastening nails and picture hooks, vacuum cleaner bags, etc., you want to know they're there when you need them. So buy back-ups. And put them where you can find them quickly.

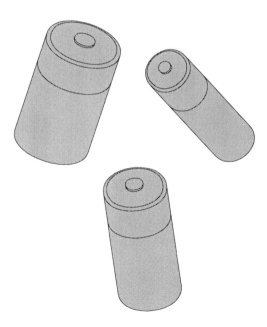

Security Away from Home

What's the most important security device you should have ...outside your home?

A cell phone.

Repeat a cell phone.

Let's begin with an emergency. The emergency number worldwide for a mobile phone is 112. Even if keypad is locked, this number can still be dialed.

Even if you're out of the coverage area of your mobile network and there is an emergency, the mobile will search any existing network to establish an emergency number for you.

It can also come through for you in tough situations. For instance, if your car has remote keyless entry, and you're in a panic mode because you locked the car and can't find your keys, the car can still be unlocked. CHECK SECTION ON DID YOU KNOW?

Calling Roadside Assistance? You need your cellphone, feeling safe while you wait for Roadside Assistance...thanks to your cell phone.

A cell phone can save a life...yours!

Driving on Your Own. Protect Yourself.

Beyond keeping your cell phone close at hand, there are other ways to keep yourself safe from harm's way. For instance, take care where you park staying clear of unlit areas and places where few cars are parked. Lock your car and be sure to mark down where you are parked, i.e. parking level 3, space 14G.

When you return to your parking space, check out someone sitting in a vehicle parked next to you. Bad guys could easily hang out there. Unsure? Get help. The adage: If you see something, say something is the right message here.

Have your keys ready. Criminals only need a few seconds to act. And LOCK your car immediately once you get in.

Pulled over by an unmarked "police car"? If you don't think you've done something wrong, call 911; they can tell you if it's legitimate or not. Still not sure? Continue to a more populated area like a gas station or convenience store. Ask for ID; we're told that police doing traffic patrol use unmarked cars, but rarely are they out of uniform.

Keep your car well serviced. That applies for car batteries, especially in cold weather. Tires need to be checked and rotated. Emergencies call for fast action. Having your car well maintained can help you avoid trouble later on. (See chapter on Regular Check-ups for your car and his.)

Another Feel Good Page

Now's the time to give yourself a pat on the back for doing what HE used to do, fixing what he used to fix, mastering the big and little jobs he used to master.

We're proud of you. And YOU should be proud of YOU, too.

Safety Deposit Box vs.
Hiding Valuables Under Your Undies

Most likely, HE took charge of safekeeping. The stock certificates, the jewelry, the titles to the cars, the wills, and sometimes, seeking a safe place for the family silver. All of the items that are extremely valuable and often difficult to replace.

Consider, if YOU haven't one, a safety deposit box at your local bank. Some offer small ones free if you have an account there. And if they charge for a box, the fee is a modest one. In it should be valuable papers like life, home, car, and health insurance policies, home mortgage, land titles, stock certificates along with jewelry, and other valuables that are irreplaceable.

Keep a list of contents along with the keys. The bank gives you two keys. Label the keys with box number and name of bank. AS DISCUSSED BEFORE, keep your safety deposit keys in the place you designated for safekeeping.

Note: Banks consolidate, change their name, and even go out of business. KEEP UP TO DATE WHICH FINANCIAL INSTITUTION HOLDS YOUR SAFETY DEPOSIT BOX. THINGS CAN FALL THROUGH THE CRACKS.

Do NOT keep your will in the safety deposit box. This belongs in the file with other financial papers.

Protecting Your Privacy: Get a Shredder

Yes, HE was keeper of the books. The financial heavy. Now YOU have to pick up where HE left off. And, perhaps, make some improvements.

First step, a simple one, but a necessary one: Buy a shredder if you don't already own one. Protecting your records, your privacy and your identity today can be a full time job. An inexpensive shredder can ensure your security when it comes to JUNK MAIL, special "offers", false solicitations and other scams.

Next, when one of those solicitations for a new credit card, complete with an offer to give you bonus frequent flyer miles, comes in the mail, don't bother to open the envelope. Shred it and the card enclosed in the shredder. You probably get one of these offers once a week. Shred it!

Shredders are also useful for the dozens of coupons, charity letters, junk mail that fills your mail box each and every day.

AND IF YOU do open some of the "junk" mail, do not be taken in by what seem to be on the surface FREE offers. Read the fine print. Ninety-nine times out of 100, there is a catch!

Pin Numbers, Passwords
and Other Secret Stuff

When there were TWO of YOU, HE may have been the one writing checks, paying the bills, handling the day to day financials. That required establishing passwords and pin numbers for each account, be it line of credit, charge and/or debit account, brokerage, internet service, frequent flyer account, etc.

Now it's YOUR responsibility. We suggest first, take it slow. Make a list of all the institutions you will be dealing with. Then, choose a pin number—the same pin number for as many as possible. It's usually six digits. Keep this list of pin numbers in that same drawer where you keep extra car keys, keys to the safety deposit box, extra house keys.

Be aware that today banks and other credit institutions are extremely careful releasing information over the phone. Some require more than the last 4 digits of your social security number. Be prepared with answers to mother's maiden name, place of birth, address where you lived as a child, favorite color, and so forth. Consider asking for a phone number so you can check out if call is legitimate.

Tip: Hide-a-key "rocks" are easy finds for burglars. DON'T hide your front door key there.

Tip: Don't give out your S.S. number unless you've thoroughly checked out caller. Too many scams going on today.

Note: CHECK OUT CHAPTER ON SCAMS. Today it's vital to know your enemy.

SCAMS!
HE seemed to smell them out.
YOU need to be prepared.

And believe me they happen. We've all had occasion to receive the telephone call, with a believable, best friend voice trying to sell us home security protection, lower rates for insurance, long term health care, help with taxes and handling the estate, and so on. The internet is full of them. PLUS Mail with bonus offers. Mail with scare tactics. Official government letters. E-mail, even pre-screened e-mail.

Too often, we fall prey to these unscrupulous characters. No matter how much you try to screen the calls, THEY get through.

We urge you to take a deep breath, inhale and exhale, and get on with YOUR life. As you will come to realize, 100% are scams offered up by con artists who have "brilliant", can't miss deals that will double, triple your investment. Sure.

And if HE was the one who handled the finances, you were lucky. HE dealt with the solicitations, and fortunately for you was able to fend off the bad guys, the scam artists. Women are the main prey of these scam artists. Widows and divorcees head the list.

What can YOU do?

BEWARE. BE ALERT THAT THE SCAM-ERS ARE OUT THERE. SO, IF YOU GET A CALL THAT DOESN'T SEEM TOTALLY HONEST, OR EVEN HALF WAY HONEST, BE SURE YOU DO NOT DIVULGE ANY PERSONAL INFORMATION, I.E. SOCIAL SECURITY NUMBER, LAST 4 DIGITS OF CREDIT CARDS, MOTHER'S MAIDEN NAME, SCHOOLS YOU ATTENDED. REFUSE TO PROVIDE ANY INFORMATION. AND THEN, HANG UP!

Basic Overview:
Handling Money Matters on Your Own

Whether you're a divorcee, widow, or the one whose significant other is no longer significant, YOU are now faced with handling money matters on your own. This goes for changing ownership on insurance policies: auto, home, annuities, etc. You may decide to name new beneficiaries, change the coverage you have, etc.

Same goes for medical insurance, long term health care, bank accounts, particularly joint accounts, stocks and bonds, land titles, annuities, credit cards, anything and everything you owned or paid for together. You need to take a long look at what you own yourself, what you own together, and what are the next steps you need to consider for ensuring a safe and comfortable future. For YOU. For YOUR family.

This does not have to be accomplished in one day. Take your time. And get help if you need it. (SEE chapter on Financial Advisors.)

If YOU're a widow, make sure YOU get all the widow's benefits.

Often, the emotional side of loss and widowhood clouds our thinking about the financial, numbers side. Go slowly here.

Whether you decide to handle your finances yourself or to use a financial guru, it's important to review what survivor benefits you may be eligible for, i.e. HIS Social Security, veteran's benefits, life insurance, employer provided health insurance, HIS IRA account. YOU owe it to yourself to get the full benefit for all the years YOU and HE were together.

How to take HIS name off what is now YOUR car, YOUR checkbook, YOUR credit card accounts, etc.

Now's the time to get real about the fact that HE'S no longer in your life. And HIS name should be dropped from anything you co-owned.

That goes for car registration, car insurance, joint bank accounts, credit cards joint brokerage accounts, joint everything.

Let's start with the car: Rather than deal with the bureaucracy of a personal encounter with the Motor Vehicle Department, go on line to get specific information for your state. This way, you'll be prepared before you go to the MVD.

Now visit your local MVD. Be patient. Despite prepping yourself before hand, you may need additional paper work.

Keep your cool. You will succeed ultimately.

As for bank and brokerage accounts, if you are a widow, you will need copies of the death certificate, and depending upon the bank or brokerage house, additional proof of yourself as beneficiary.

Today, with all the scams, financial houses are overly careful. This can take time. But YOU will prevail.

The scenario may be easier if you and HE split, legally or otherwise. Most likely, going to your local bank or financial security office and filling out forms will take care of this. But again, today, banks and brokerage houses are paranoid about scams.

BE PATIENT!

Note: HIS name may not show on bank statements; check this out carefully just in case he is listed with the bank.

Other details to be aware of: Changing ownership on insurance policies such as auto, home? This also may mean changing beneficiaries. Check this out with the parent companies. Most include websites and/or telephone numbers on their bills or policies.

Medical insurance? If he was in a group, see if you can continue. This can save you money so it's worth checking into.

This can be a long, sometimes difficult process. Stay with it. You may find YOU're on the receiving end of some extra dollars.

Stop, look listen to some handy, gosh I wish I'd known that, tips for coping with everyday household tasks — the ones HE helped with.

Did you know that ....

Never painted a wall before? Consider this before you pick up a brush: DID YOU KNOW THAT if you put flat paint over gloss or semi gloss you're doing a no no?? It won't work, doesn't stick very well. If you really want a no shine to the paint, then you are going to have to do a light sandpaper job first. Ask your trusty hardware store about details. By the way, gloss or semi gloss over flat is no problem.

Tired of lugging that unwieldy and heavy laundry basket to the basement? DID YOU KNOW THAT there is an easier way? Stuff the items to be laundered in a big plastic garbage bag and drag it down the basement stairs. Lots lighter, easier, and you get one free hand to hold the railing. If you live in an apartment that free hand comes in handy (!) for the elevator button. No matter what, the bag thing is lots easier to deal with.

If you're like me, every time you come home from the grocery store with umpteen bags from weekly shopping YOU remember how your guy used to come out to help carry. Gone are those days! DID YOU KNOW THAT there is another helping hand available? Get a cart with wheels. Stuff as many bags as possible into it, and you've saved umpty-ump trips over the year.

So maybe YOUR guy was the one who handled the breakfast chore and now you're scrambling solo to do the eggs et al. But are they fresh? And, two, are they the ones you hard boiled the other day or not? Bet you can't remember! Let's begin with how to tell if they're fresh: DID YOU KNOW THAT if you put the eggs in a bowl of water, the outdated ones will rise to the top (throw these away), the fresh ones will stay on the bottom and the so-so ones will turn on end and float around the middle somewhere?

If your eggs didn't make it to the top, next time store them on the bottom shelf of your refrigerator. It's the coldest spot in the fridge.

Hard boiled or not? DID YOU KNOW how simple it is to find out? Spin the egg. A raw one tries to spin but wobbles, a soft-boiled egg tries to spin but will not succeed, while a hard-boiled one spins rapidly on its end. Try it next time YOU draw a blank.

Bet HE marked his eggs with date of purchase. YOU should, too.

Frustrated trying to open the sticky drawer that HE always opened 1-2-3? You tug and tug, and it stays stuck. DID YOU KNOW THAT WD-40, that blue can with the funny name HE kept in the broom closet, can solve the problem in a jiffy? Just spray along drawer opening. Drawer should open easily.

Note: Check chapters on fixing things inside the house for other helpful suggestions.

Locked out of your car? DID YOU KNOW THAT if you have a keyless key to your car, and you've locked your car, and can't find the keys (probably somewhere between the shopping center or grocery store and the spare keys are at home, you can still unlock your car long distance. Use your cell phone to call someone at your home on their cell phone. Once you've reached them and they've located extra set of keys, hold your cell phone a foot or so from your car door. Ask the person at your home to press the unlock button on the keyless key, holding it near the cell phone at their end. Bingo, the door lock should open. This also works for the trunk lock. WE BET HE DIDN'T KNOW THIS. NOW YOU'RE ONE UP ON HIM.

Note: The website, Snopes, questioned this. Other sites claim it does work.

If HE was the designated driver, and YOU were the navigator, getting to your destination was a team effort. Now that you're on your own, get yourself up to date, detailed road maps, (triple AAA is an excellent source), and invest in a GPS. It's money well spent for peace of mind on the road. And DID YOU KNOW that you can use the GPS for locating street addresses? The ones you can unplug can be carried on the street to locate a store, restaurant, friend's home, etc. Nifty in an unfamiliar city.

What to do when you've lost your cell somewhere in YOUR very own house? Sounds DUHHH, but when you're desperate to find the cell phone, JUST call yourself on your land phone. YOU do know where that is. (HE would have thought of that in a nanosecond.} No land phone? C'mon, try a neighbor's! Now if finding YOUR misplaced eyeglasses could only be this easy.

DID YOU KNOW that there is a worldwide emergency number for your mobile phone? 112. If you're out of the coverage area of your mobile network, and there is an emergency, dial 112. You will be connected to local emergency contact even if you are outside your provider's service area. It works even if keypad is locked. Bet HE didn't know that either.

Note: As one would expect, "glitches" happen and in remote areas of the world, you may not get through.

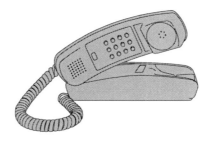

General Advice: Splitting the Bill

You're out to dinner with two couples, and the check arrives. What now?

An uncomfortable moment. We guarantee that one guy will say to the other, "Let's treat her; we'll just split it down the middle" This is YOUR opportunity to become a noose around your friends' necks… or to look them straight in the eye, smile, and say, "You're both so great, but I really do want to pay my own way. Thanks."

Immediately follow this little speech by putting your credit card in front of them. Done! The next time you go out with married friends, it will be "de rigeur." And there will be a next time. Because now they can enjoy your company without figuring how much it may cost them.

Tip #1. What should you leave the wait staff? Fifteen to 20% is pretty much the standard today. Remember to just tip on the food and drink part of the bill. Not the Total Bill after tax has been added. There's nothing cheap about this. It is the correct thing to do.

Tip #2. In some parts of the country, doubling the tax works out perfectly. (And it's so easy to do).

Making Travel Arrangements
(Have Suitcase...Will Travel)

Booking trips is a task MOST MEN TAKE ON HAPPILY. After all, they are Masters of the Universe. They also have Administrative Assistants they can call upon to execute their orders.

Now that task is YOURS. And it doesn't have to be a daunting one.

First of all, YOU have several alternatives.

> **1.** You can delegate this responsibility to a travel agent. And plenty of them are knowledgeable and helpful. Here, friend, know that it's in your best interest to be COMPLETELY straightforward, giving them an idea of budget, time of year you choose to travel, type of trip you are interested in. The more information you give them, the easier for them to find a trip that suits you.

> **2.** You can search the internet for information on packaged tours, traveling alone tours, special interest tours, budget tours, the possibilities are almost endless. I highly recommend doing this. I've taken dozens of trips as a single, and have been disappointed only once.

> I had a romantic vision of St. Petersberg Russia...a Dr. Zhivago version with Omar Sharif, the sleigh, the furs, the dazzling lights, the whole nine yards. Reality fell short of this version. Very short. There was no snow. There was no sleigh. There was no Omar Sharif. Just a very old Russian lady selling postcards for outrageous amounts of money at the Kremlin.

> But 9 times out of 10, in today's computer age, the internet is the best route to pursue if you have the time and patience.

> **3.** You can stay home and travel via the movies or TV or National Geographic.

In today's market, and with the increased sophistication of the internet search engines, we heartily recommend using internet sourcing and booking.

How to Stop Writing all those
Checks Every Month: No catch!

It's simple. Ask the companies that bill you monthly to withdraw what you owe from your checking account every month. It's called automatic withdrawal or direct debiting. Once you set this up, (which is no big deal to do), you'll wonder why you didn't do it sooner.

You'll save time by not writing those checks, and balancing your checkbook is easier (less things to write down incorrectly and less mistakes subtracting), and no stamps to buy. The bucks you save on postage alone will get you a very nice "free" lunch once a year.

This method of payment can be set up with practically every bank, saving and loan and credit union in the United States. Here's how to do it: Call the billing department where you have your car loan, your credit card provider, phone company, cable company, etc. Tell them you want to pay your bill by having the money automatically withdrawn from your account each month. Give them the name and address of your bank, the ABA routing number (the nine digit number found at bottom left corner of check) and your account number. They may also ask for a voided check and an authorization signed by you.

Note: Banks differ in what they require for automatic withdrawals, but the total process is quite simple.

And don't forget that even though you're not writing checks, you still must deduct the automatic debits done monthly from your check book balance.

Many, many young people use this method to pay their bills. Could it be that some times our kids ARE smarter than we are?

The ABC's of the ATM

No more waiting in long teller lines. It's a snap to get and use an ATM card. Just go to your bank branch and request one. (They're free). The first thing the bank officer will want you to do is to select a PIN number. A PIN is what assures you security. No one, no one, knows it but you. Once you enter that number into the machine, the ATM knows you're you and it's safe to give you cash.

Here, step by step, is how to work the machine. It is very user friendly. Mine even asks, "Do you need more time?" If I'm being pokey, I just press the Yes button and proceed at my own pace.

There are ATM machines all over the world. Besides getting dollars in the USA, you can get Euros in Paris, yen in Tokyo, you get the picture. What's the cost of a transaction? Often, none if you use your own bank's ATM.

A few important words of warning: It's easy to forget to put the amount of the withdrawal in your checkbook record. Do it while you're away or make a note of it so it's recorded when you return home. AND ALWAYS, remember to take your card with you after you've picked up your cash.

Do NOT divulge your pin number to anyone but your bank.

> **Tip:** Don't assume the ATM closes when the bank does. It's available 24/7. What a joy!

> **Tip:** Don't use an obvious pin like your dog's name or your birthday. Someone with fraud on their mind will come up with that one.

> **Tip:** Once you have a pin number, be consistent with as many as you can, using the same pin number for the bank vault, the house alarm, etc. Otherwise, remembering which is which can be a little difficult. Trust us!

IMPORTANT FINAL TIP: See chapters on Pin Numbers, Passwords and other secret stuff, Scams for further help.

A Free Flight to Paris, YOURS for the Asking

Perhaps at this moment the idea doesn't appeal to you. Your husband has just died — or your guy has walked — and what fun could a trip possibly be without your true love?

Understandable, but trust us, one day you WILL want to get away. So why not travel for next to nothing?

YOU can if you are a widow. Not so, alas, if your man was your "partner". The secret to the freebee is to simply transfer your late husband's frequent flyer miles into one single account, yours.

Easy as 1,2,3. Listen up and act now. Because most airlines have time limits.

AMERICAN AIRLINES

1. Call their toll-free number: 800-882-8880 and request the transfer.

2. They will send you a form asking for your husband's death certificate, your Advantage number and his, and your credit card information. For...uh-oh... a $50 transfer fee. Yes, we did call this deal "free", but you must admit it's almost free!.

3. Mail all this, along with your address to: American Airlines, PO Box 619688, DFW Airport, Texas 75261. Once you apply, the miles will be in your account within two to three weeks. IMPORTANT TO NOTE: If the account has been inactive (no credit card or flight activity) for 18 months, American takes back miles. Check your husband's monthly American statement to determine cut-off date. Once miles become yours, you have 18 months to redeem them. As long as there is activity, time is extended. BON VOYAGE!

U.S. AIRWAYS

1. Call their toll-free number at 800-428-4322

2. They will ask you to send your husband's death certificate, his dividend miles number plus your name, address and account number.

3. Mail to U.S. AIRWAYS Dividend Miles, PO Box 20050, Phoenix, Arizona 85036. There is no charge.

UNITED

1. Call them at 800-241-6522, toll free.

2. Rather than call, if you prefer, you can write them at: PO Box 6120, Rapid City, South Dakota 57709. They will need your husband's name, and Mileage Plus Number for both of you. They will also request a death certificate. Also include your name and address.

3. $75 charge. Give them your credit card number. They also request your e-mail address. PLEASE NOTE: Miles expire in 18 months. Apply during that time frame, and once in your account, you have 18 months to use. Credit card activity using a United Mileage card will extend that time.

SOUTHWEST

Their Rapid Rewards ARE transferable. Call this number, unfortunately it's not toll-free, 214/792-4223. Hours are 8 to 5, Central Time. We hope you have better luck than we did getting through to them. Keep trying.

Check out their website: www.SouthwestAirlines.com that has everything BUT information about transferring miles upon a death. Maybe by the time you read this, they will be up to speed. Let's hope so.

JET BLUE

Has no direct phone line to their True Blue program. However, you can reach mileage department by calling Jet Blue's regular number (toll free: 800-538-2523) and a representative will transfer you over. At this writing, it is a half hour wait due to surge of people wanting to book using their miles or asking questions about changes in the program. Currently, miles are not transferrable. To find out whether an exception is made in the event of death, we were told we had to speak to someone in that department. We didn't get through. Worth checking out just in case they've changed their policy and do transfer miles.

CONTINENTAL

1. Call them at their toll free number 713-952-1630

2. Continental would like a copy of HIS death certificate and his will if in it he has bequeathed his mileage to you. If not, Continental will provide you with a "hold harmless" legal form to sign. They will also want "One Pass" Account numbers for YOU and your late husband. Send along with your address to One Pass Service Center, PO Box 4365, Houston, North Carolina 77210-4365.

3. Transfer takes two weeks. There is no fee. Miles do not expire, lucky you, so you can wait as long as you like to request the transfer, and once you get it, to use your miles. We urge you to use the miles quickly as airlines today are here today, gone tomorrow.

DELTA

1. Call them at 800-221-1212, toll-free number.

2. Delta will want a copy of the death certificate, frequent flyer number for your husband, your photo ID, e-mail address and account information (name, address, frequent flyer number). Send to Delta Airlines, Dept. 654, PO Box 20532, Atlanta, Georgia 30320-2532. Or fax to: 404/773-1945.

3. No fee. If no activity (flights or frequent flyer credit card) within a two year period, you lose the miles.

Authors' P.S.

This book is a generous helping of suggestions on how to do what HE used to do around the house. How to fix what he used to fix...now that he's gone. We wrote it because we realize there are lots — thousands — of women out there in the same place as you. Looking for answers, a helping hand, and a pat on the back for a job well done.

No, you can't have HIS help, but YES YOU CAN find your way through the ups and downs of being on your own. GOOD LUCK. And do keep in touch.

love, lainey and ollie

The End.

No, the beginning of a new life. A fuller, richer life, on your own.

Our hearts and hopes are with you.

lainey and ollie

Index

NOTES:

Keep these pages FOR MAKING NOTE OF tips, ideas, short cuts, critical phone numbers, etc. that YOU discover doing the things HE used to do.

NOTES:

NOTES:

NOTES: